AN OSTEOPATH`S GUIDE TO NUTRITION

A to Z of Vitamins, Minerals, Herbs
& Food Supplements

Rohan Iswariah D.O.

Copyright © 2022 Rohan Iswariah

Copyright © 2022 Rohan Iswariah All rights reserved

No part of this book may be reproduced, except for the information already available in the public domain, or stored in a retrieval system, or transmitted in any form or by any means, electronic, mechanical, photocopying, recording, or otherwise, without express written permission of the publisher.

Disclaimer Notice:

Although the author and publisher have made every effort to ensure the information in this book was correct at time of going to press, the author and publisher do not assume and hereby disclaim any liability to any party for any loss, damage, or disruption caused by errors or omissions, whether such errors or omissions result from negligence, accident, or any other cause. This book is not intended as a substitute for the medical advice of physicians and is not intended to provide diagnosis or treatment advice. The reader should regularly consult a physician in matters relating to his/her health and particularly with respect to any symptoms that may require a professional diagnosis and/or medical attention.

This book is affectionately dedicated to my wife Jane and my children Freddie & Amelia. Also gratefully acknowledged is the invaluable inspiration given to me by Karen, Klair, Penny, both Pats & Louises & many of my patients, without whom this book could not have been written.

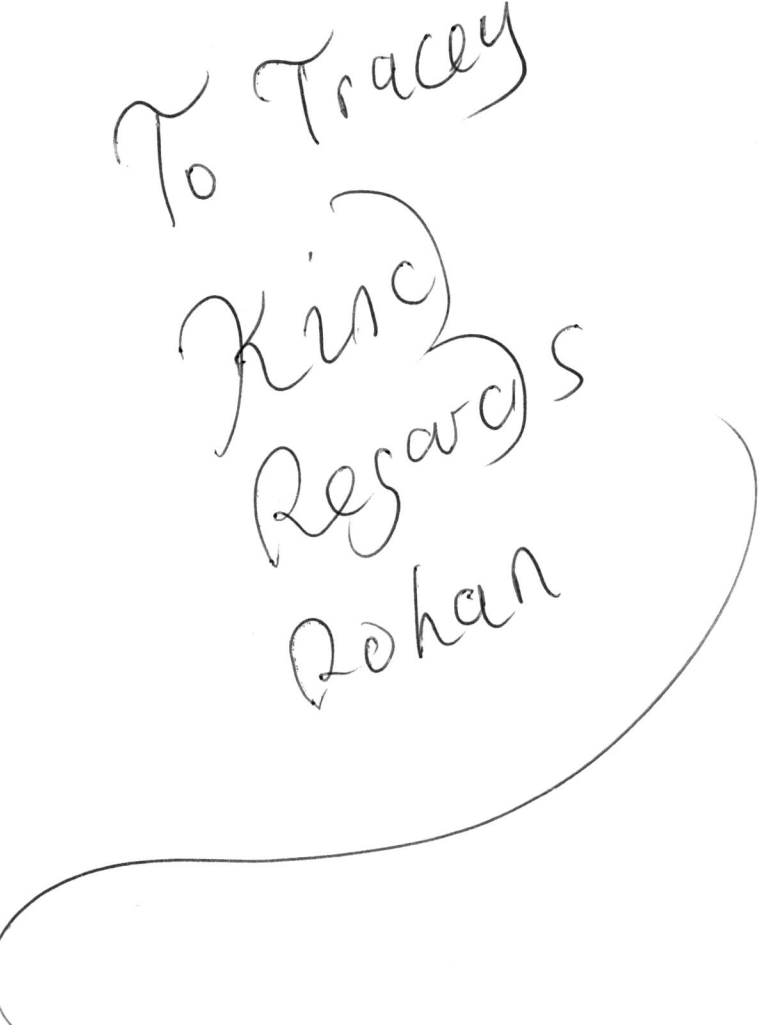

CONTENTS

Title Page
Copyright
Dedication
Preface 1
Introduction 2
A 31
B 44
C 62
D 81
E 87
F 93
G 100
H 109
I 114
J 117
K 119
L 123
M 130
N 141
O 144
P 148

Q	159
R	161
S	164
T	171
U	175
V	176
W	178
X	180
Y	181
Z	184
Conclusion	187

PREFACE

I have been an osteopath for over 38 years since qualifying from The British School of Osteopathy in 1983. As an osteopath I recognise that many factors can cause or contribute to ill health. Osteopaths try to provide a whole-person approach to health, and use various techniques tailored to the individual to achieve or provide effective care and treatment. Patients will often discuss a host of factors that can illuminate the cause of their presenting symptoms - nutrition can be one of these. As osteopaths take a holistic approach to promoting well-being and preventing disease, where possible, good nutrition is a vital factor that assists in healthy functioning. Good nutrition is vital for growth, providing energy, gut health, building and maintaining the immune system, and contributes to proper digestion. It protects us against many chronic noncommunicable diseases, such as heart disease, diabetes, and cancer. Good nutrition is also important for maintaining our memory and contributes to good mood. I wrote this book to appraise all the vitamins and minerals, and many food supplements by using as many authoritative papers as I could find, so that the reader could be better informed when looking for supplements, when appropriate, and might be armed with information to ask further questions.

INTRODUCTION

This book is organised for the convenience of the reader in an A-to-Z format that tries to investigate the health benefits derived from vitamins, minerals, food supplements, various herbs, and compounds. The book can be used as a reference guide, if the reader wishes to dip in-and-out, and can be used to follow the references further if desired. For example, if there is a news item about vitamins D or E, or an article in a newspaper concerning lithium, the reader can access additional information under the relevant chapter heading and entry, which is placed in alphabetical order. Entries could relate to the historical discovery, current and traditional uses, and where appropriate, the recommended dietary allowances, or adequate intakes, and upper tolerable limits; these relate to all vitamins and minerals, and some other entries too. I have tried to access as many abstracts, papers, websites, and other sources as possible, and have referenced these in the individual entries, which are available as endnotes — additionally, some useful websites are listed at the back of the book for further reading and exploration. I wanted to both educate myself and inform others and have come across some interesting and sometimes surprising facts whilst compiling this book. In this introduction I have tried to give the reader some additional information to give individual entries context and hopefully "whet the appetite" further!

Plants and Herbs

Plants and herbs are — and have been — used across all continents, historically forming the basis of all folk and traditional holistic medical systems. Originating in India over 3,000 years ago, and maybe more than 5,000 years, is the ancient medical system known as Ayurveda. Generations of Indian people gathered medical knowledge, largely through experience, which was then passed on, orally in the beginning, and then compiled in a canon of sacred records; this literature is known as the Vedas. The Chinese are believed to have studied most of these Sanskrit texts many centuries ago, and this has almost certainly informed Traditional Chinese Medicine (TCM). TCM also uses a variety of plants and Chinese herbs — and is over 3,500 years old itself. Plants and herbs (herbs are described as any plant that has a medicinal or food usage for humans or animals) have been used to ease or cure maladies for many thousands of years, with uses predating recorded history itself.

Many of our modern prescription drugs originate from plants. Two examples are aspirin, originally derived from willow bark, and yohimbine hydrochloride, extracted from Yohimbe (an evergreen plant species that is native to western and central Africa). The celebrated active ingredient obtained from the willow tree, or shrub, is salicylic acid — a phytohormone also found in numerous other plants. Phytohormones are known plant growth regulators and active compounds produced by plants in response to stress. In humans, salicylic acid (aspirin) is used as a medication to reduce fever and inflammation, relieve pain, and as a blood thinning agent. Phytohormones also play a role in plant development, assisting with ion uptake and transportation, transpiration, and photosynthesis. Most plants contain salicylic acid or other derivatives, such as salicin, or methyl salicylates — to both protect themselves from harmful pathogens, and to fulfil some of the above roles. Some of these plants are described within this book. Other plant derived compounds used in modern medicines are digoxin (from the foxglove), which is used to control some heart problems, quinine (from cinchona bark), a medication used to treat malaria and babesiosis (babesiosis is a rare and life-threatening infection of the red blood cells spread by ticks. Babesia microti is the parasitic blood-borne kind that affects humans, which is carried by deer ticks), and morphine, a strong painkiller isolated from the opium poppy.[1] A 2020 review of plant phytochemicals such as flavonoids, tannins, saponins, and alkaloids showed beneficial inhibitory effects for humans in peptic ulcer disease (PUD) — a condition caused by an infection from the Helicobacter pylori bacterium. The same review also concluded that medicinal plants from both the Asteraceae or Compositae (with over 32,000 species of flowering plants),[2] and Fabaceae families (with in excess of 20,000 species of trees, shrubs, vines, and herbs worldwide)[3] have been shown to be effective, safe and widely available alternative therapeutics for several other diseases, including PUD.[4] Wild plants and flowers are the sources of most folk medicines or ethno-medicines across the world. These are not genetically modified in the same way as some of our ornamental flowers and plants are nowadays, and therefore retain much of their original code. Wild plants don`t tend to need watering either!

Plants contain a tremendous number of compounds that fulfil self-protective functions and provide disease resistance from pathogens. These are known as phytochemicals (Fight-Oh!). These protective chemicals are preformed structures or compounds, but plants also have a type of two-branched immune system, with both an innate generalised response to the molecules common to many classes of microbes, and a more specific one, an infection induced response that can move from cell to cell through the plant`s vascular system. The vascular system of a plant consists of an assemblage of conducting tissues and associated supporting structures. (The xylem transports water and dissolved minerals to the leaves, and the phloem conducts food from the leaves to the whole of the plant).[5] However, this immune response differs from mammals, as plants do not have circulating immune cells — as we do — in our blood. The first response to invasion is the more non-specific one and represents a broader range of antimicrobial defences exhibited by most plant cell types. The very first line of defence plants often use is a thick bark or a waxy cuticle that repels physical invasion from pathogens and animals (mainly herbivores). Plants are very nutritious to a wide range of animals, which includes humans of course, and therefore need to protect themselves, unless ingestion serves another vital purpose, such as the propagation of their own seeds. Many seeds (also known as stones, pits, and kernels) contain amygdalin that breaks down into hydrogen cyanide (a poisonous compound) — animals often excrete the seeds for this reason, which keeps the seeds viable (this ingestion process of dispersal is known as endozoochory). Whilst plants do not have a nervous system, some can emit compounds that alert others to approaching threats. A bit like a human shouting out, "Watchout" or "Run". However, plants cannot run away, so specific chemical profiles represent their main self-protective weapons. Various other methods of plant protection have evolved over many millions of years, with some plants possessing thorns, prickles, and spines — such as roses and cacti — to ward off consumers. Nettles, for example, have the capacity to sting the unwary; the compounds responsible are formic acid and histamine. The latter chemical is the reason that rubbing a nettle sting with a dock leaf can help relieve the burning, itching, redness, and swelling, as dock leaf sap contains a natural antihistamine, which helps to relieve the associated stinging sensation. Others, like Dumb canes, which are flowering plants native to the New World Tropics, house pain-inducing chemicals in razor-sharp crystals called raphides (Oxalate compounds). Please do not consume this plant — it is just for ornamental enjoyment! Another example of an edible plant that contains a similar chemical defence is rhubarb, which has oxalic acid in its leaves, a compound that is toxic to most animals. Some plants that contain little defence of their own will recruit others to assist. For example, the African acacia tree houses aggressive ants, which protect the plant from herbivores, and in turn, the tree provides nectar and other nutrients to the ants. The term for this beneficial relationship for both parties is mutualism, and this evolved ecological partnership between different species is a commonly used strategy in the plant and animal kingdom. Some plants will feign dead by closing their leaves, others may even release compounds that attract the enemy`s predators themselves. Research has shown plants can communicate approaching dangers with each other. This communication can take place through root systems and fungal networks.[6] A common strategy that many plants utilise is the deployment of chemical poisons for protection. We have already mentioned the toxicity of oxalic acid and its derivative compounds to a large number of animals, and most of us are also familiar with the highly toxic nature of some mushrooms. These fungi are not for consumption, as they contain a large range of toxins, including amatoxins and muscarine. Other plants that are toxic to humans, for example, are hemlock and purple nightshade, but there are a wide variety of plants considered poisonous to us, either at different stages of their own development, or just certain parts of the plant, which may still be edible if processed properly. Some plants are selective and are only toxic to certain animals. For example, cats are extremely sensitive to alliums, the genus that includes garlic, onions, and leeks. These we humans can eat safely. However, this book is not about inedible plants. The purpose of writing about plant security is to shine a light on the reasons for these myriad methods of protection, as most plants utilise these various strategies to both survive and genetically propagate.

Homeostasis and Allostasis

In this book, the descriptions of micronutrients, which are all available in the environment for human consumption need to be appraised within the context of an individual`s personal nutritional status. This nutritional status should not be considered in isolation, as we are influenced by so many other inter-related factors. Some professions, including osteopaths, have viewed these inter-related factors, in a broad manner, by using the Bio-

Psycho-Social model, of which a representation is shown below in Fig 1.

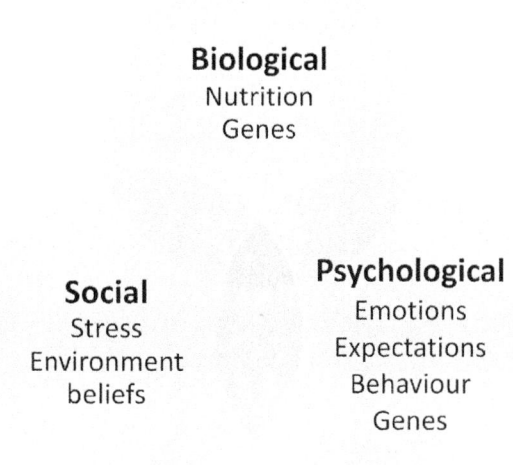

Fig 1 : Rohan Iswariah D.O. © 2020

As individuals we all need to remain in balance, and often have different requirements based upon sex, age, whether expectant or lactating in the case of women, and a host of other personal factors. This complex and often chaotic relationship is not best suited to simple cause-and-effect models. When we use the word balance, the ancient Greeks used the word homeostasis, which means — "those processes that maintain all the body systems and need to operate within narrow ranges". This can be supported by good nutrition. Some of the nutrients we consume are considered essential or conditionally essential, while others can be manufactured in the body, providing the general nutritional status or overall health of the individual is stable. A better word, in one way, than homeostasis, and also of Greek derivation, is allostasis, which refers to maintaining stability or "allostatic" balance under differing physiological circumstances and challenges presented to us, at different times of our lives.

Some examples, already briefly mentioned, are the different nutritional requirements needed during pregnancy and lactation, when in the growing phases of life, and at different ages. There are also differing requirements for males and females. Extra requirements may be necessary when fighting infections and disease too.

Nutrition

Overall, a balanced diet containing sufficient nutritional elements is critical for health, and both nutritional deficiencies and excesses can be associated with disease.[7] The following diagram (please see Fig 2) shows several important factors that can affect the individual, including good balanced nutrition; all the factors are inter-related and can influence the overall health status of a person.

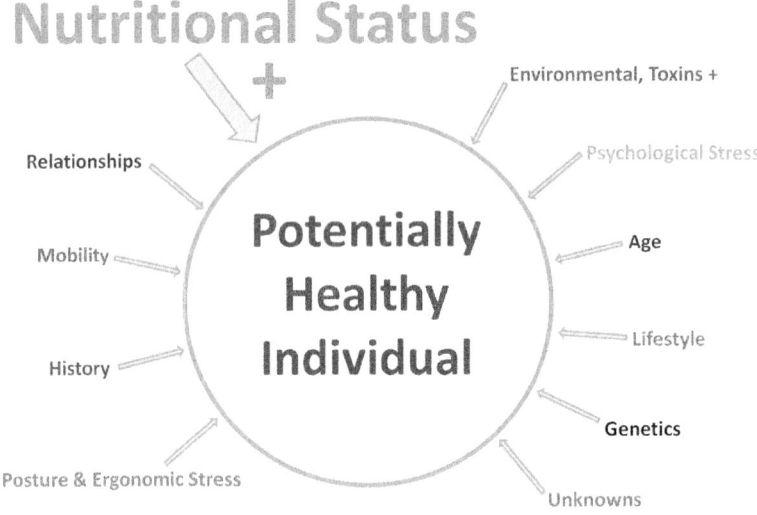

Fig 2 : Rohan Iswariah D.O. © 2020

A negative nutritional status can also affect different people in various ways. The World Health Organization describes malnutrition as deficiencies, excesses, or imbalances in a person's intake of energy and/or nutrients; and malnutrition addresses three broad groups.

- Undernutrition, which includes wasting (low weight-for-height), stunting (low height-for-age) and underweight (low weight-for-age)
- Micronutrient-related malnutrition, which includes micronutrient deficiencies (a lack of important vitamins and minerals) or micronutrient excess; and
- Overweight, which leads to obesity and various diet-related non-communicable diseases (these include heart disease, stroke, diabetes, and some cancers).

Malnutrition is a major cause, or contributor, involved with the prevalence of many diseases and syndromes, such as Marasmus and Kwashiorkor, including symptoms such as lethargy, tiredness, irritability, depression, poor wound healing, weight loss, and developmental problems. In a way, and at the other end of the scale, is overeating, which causes obesity and consequentially increases the risks of diet-related non-communicable diseases. These include cardiovascular disease, type 2 diabetes, cancer, and metabolic syndrome. Malnutrition also includes vitamin and mineral deficiencies that can contribute to osteoporosis and anaemia, for example. Malnutrition particularly affects children and pregnant women in low-income countries. The World Health Organization (WHO) estimates that globally 1.9 billion adults are obese and 462 million are underweight. In 2020 WHO also estimated that 45 million children under 5 years of age were wasted and 149 million were stunted, while 38.9 million children were considered overweight or obese; and these extremes coexisted at the same time and in the same countries,[8] (please see Fig 3 below). Good nutrition, for everyone, can only be solved globally through international cooperation, education, and coherent government policies?[9]

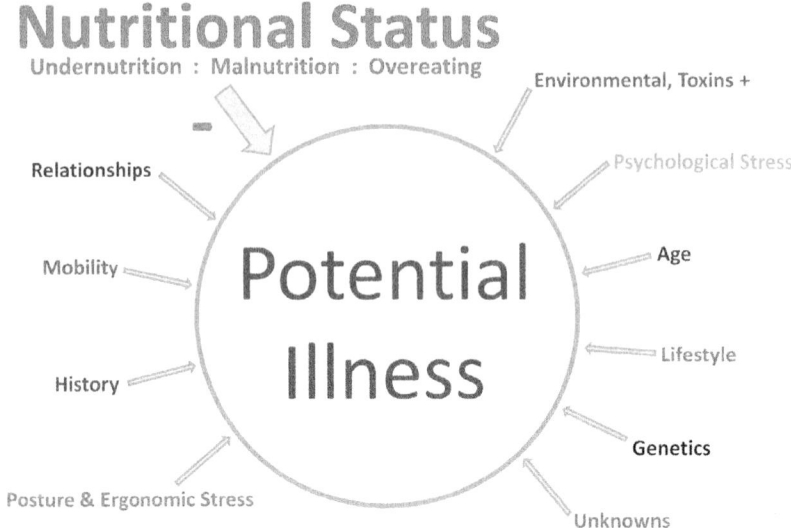

Fig 3 : Rohan Iswariah D.O. © 2020

Productivity

The rate of growth in agricultural productivity is declining globally. This presents a problem with respect to the number of hectares of land that will be required to feed and support a growing population. The diagram below (please see Fig 4) uses a conservative or median figure to estimate the world population in 2050, and this shows that between 6 and 6.4 people will need to be supported by a single hectare of land; in 1960 this figure was approximately 2.4 people per hectare, when the global population was only around 3 billion.

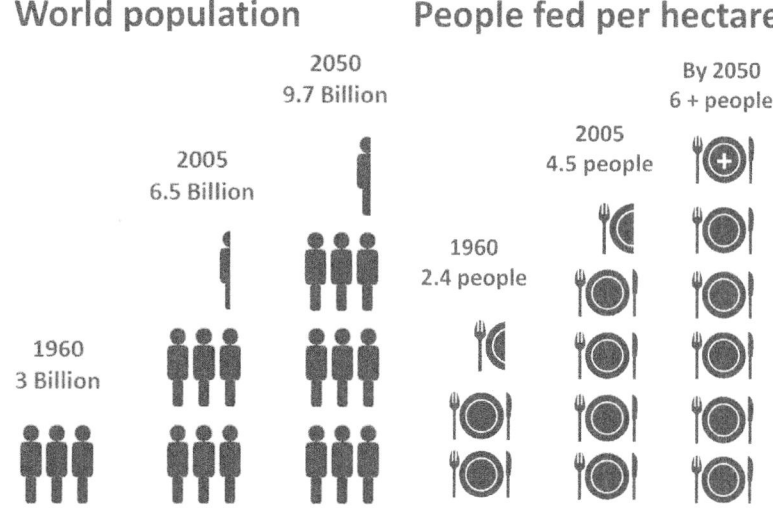

Data sources: United Nations projections in 2019, FAO.org, WorldBank.org   Fig 4 : Rohan Iswariah D.O. © 2020

The declining productivity growth rate is thought in part to be due to the over-reliance of farmers on increasing the levels of inputs, such as fertilisers and pesticides, to increase production. This harms the soils and delicate ecosystems, consequently bringing diminishing returns.[10] Climate change is another increasingly important factor affecting productivity. All of these factors mean a wide spectrum of solutions will be required to ensure good nutrition for people across the whole world, in the not-too-distant future. Another different set of problems are considered influential for nutritional status, which relate to possible declining fertility rates, also presenting demographic challenges. These are not related directly to productivity itself.

Food Supplements

Food supplements are described in EU law as, "any food the purpose of which is to supplement the normal diet and which is a concentrated source of a vitamin, or mineral, or other substance with a nutritional or physiological effect, alone or in combination, and sold in dose form."[11] They are all regulated in the UK under the provisions of general food law.[12]

Antioxidants

Antioxidants are a wide-ranging group of different compounds that may help to protect body cells from free radical damage. Free radicals are types of unstable molecules that are made during normal metabolism (all the chemical reactions that take place within each cell of a living organism). Free radicals can build up in our cells and cause damage to other molecules, such as DNA, lipids, and proteins. This damage is called "oxidative stress" and can increase the risk of cancer and other diseases. Some examples of natural antioxidants, include vitamins C and E, carotenoids, lycopenes, lutein, selenium, manganese, and polyphenols, such as anthocyanins. There are, in fact, more than 8,000 polyphenolic compounds that have been identified in various plant species. Apart from their antioxidant capacities, polyphenols are secondary metabolites (metabolites are intermediate or end-products of metabolism) of plants. These compounds are generally involved in plant self-defence, protecting against ultraviolet radiation, or aggression from dangerous pathogens. Oxygen is a highly reactive element that becomes incorporated in molecules. These compounds, and often oxygen itself, can be called free radicals, which are highly damaging to our own healthy cells. Our exposure to these unstable compounds and molecules is both internal and external in nature. In order to see how quickly oxidation occurs, just cut an apple in half, and you will see that it turns brown within a few minutes. This is due to the chemical reaction of the exposed apple chemicals with the oxygen present in the air. Free radicals are also formed naturally by our own metabolic processes, and occur, or appear, in the environment as airborne pollutants, such as nitrogen dioxide and sulphur dioxide, photochemicals, and cigarette smoke. Oxidative stress is thought to play a role in cancer, cardiovascular diseases, diabetes, and both Parkinson`s and Alzheimer's diseases. Oxidative stress also influences certain eye conditions, such as cataracts and age-related macular degeneration. There is good evidence to suggest eating a healthy diet, which must include lots of fruits and vegetables, lowers the risks associated with acquiring several of these diseases. Whether this is due to the quantity of antioxidants present in fruits and vegetables remains unclear, as other compounds found in these foods, lifestyle, and other factors might be implicated with benefits too. It is clear, though, that a healthy balance between free radicals and antioxidants is required for proper and efficient physiological functions to occur — thereby avoiding too much oxidative stress. A 2010 article in the publication "Pharmacognosy Review" concluded that in addition to our internal antioxidant defence systems, the consumption of dietary and plant-derived antioxidants appeared to be suitable alternatives for our own internal systems, and that both dietary and other components of plants are major sources of antioxidants.[13]

As we have seen, it is very difficult to establish exact links between health effects and the antioxidant content of any particular food type. There is not a simple "cause and effect" scenario at play here, and even measuring the actual antioxidant content of any compound has been fraught with difficulty. The antioxidant effect, for example, of an individual food substance was previously measured using a system known as the ORAC-Oxygen Radical Absorbance Capacity-. This gave certain values which were calculated in-vitro, meaning occurring outside of the living organism, as contrasted with the term in-vivo, which means taking place within the living organism. This measure, however, was not found to have sufficient scientific support in-vivo and was therefore withdrawn in 2012. So, alternative measures such as TEAC-Trolox Equivalent Antioxidant Capacity-, TRAP-Total Radical-trapping Antioxidant Parameter-, and FRAP-Ferric

Reducing Ability of Plasma- were adopted as common standards most frequently used to ascertain the general antioxidant capacity of any sample. Results, in 2010, from FRAP analysis of more than 3,100 foods, including beverages, spices, herbs, and supplements, used globally, found several thousand-fold differences in sample antioxidant capacities. Spices, herbs, and supplements were found to be the richest sources in the study. Berries, fruits, nuts, chocolate, vegetables, and certain derivative products were often found to have exceptionally high antioxidant values.[14] The human cell damage that oxidative stress and free radicals can cause is the reason antioxidants are so important, and constantly counteracting detrimental oxidative effects is considered vitally important for continuing good health.

Vitamins

There are thirteen vitamins that humans need for a variety of diverse metabolic functions. The two main groups of vitamins are basically split into two main types. There are the fat-soluble vitamins A, D, E, and K, and those vitamins which are water-soluble, vitamins B1, B2, B3, B5, B6, B7, B9, B12, and C. Previously known vitamins B4 (Adenine), B8 (Inositol), B10 (Para amino benzoic acid-PABA), and B11 (Salicylic acid) do not fit into the official definition of a vitamin. To have been defined as such would have indicated that these compounds were required in the diet, as they could not be manufactured in the human body, and therefore would have been considered essential for normal metabolism. During research into the properties of vitamins and the history of their discoveries, I discovered an interesting fact about vitamin C. As we have already seen, vitamin C is one of the thirteen vitamins that is essential to us, humans, and also some other anthropoid primates, as well as teleost fishes (members of a large and extremely diverse group of ray-finned fishes), guinea pigs, some bats, and Passeriformes (perching) bird species; all of these species have lost the capacity to synthesise vitamin C, for some ancient genetic mutational reason. Most animals, however, can make vitamin C, and it is therefore considered non-essential to them.[15]

Amino Acids

Other essential nutrients that cannot be manufactured in the human body include the essential amino acids: phenylalanine, valine, tryptophan, threonine, methionine, leucine, isoleucine, lysine, and histidine. The amino acid arginine is considered semi-essential, and for this reason is not added to the list of the nine essential amino acids. There are twenty (some postulate, twenty-one, if we include selenocysteine) amino acids, which together form all proteins, and are considered the building blocks of life, essential for growth and human function. The first amino acid was discovered in 1806 by chemists, Louis-Nicholas Vauquelin and Pierre Jean Robiquet. This compound, isolated from asparagus and named asparagine, is a non-essential amino acid, which can be synthesised in the human body.[16] The discovery of cystine by William Hyde Wollaston, also the discoverer of two elements rhodium and palladium, followed in 1810.[17] Cystine is found in many foods, including eggs, meat, dairy products, and whole grains, as well as skin, horns, and hair.[18]

Fatty Acids

There are also two essential fatty acids that cannot be made in the human body. These are alpha-linolenic acid, an omega-3 fatty acid, and linoleic acid, an omega-6 fatty acid. We will discuss the health benefits of these later in the book.

Minerals

Excluding the CHON elements — carbon, hydrogen, oxygen, and nitrogen, we also need a host of essential minerals to help growth and development, enzyme activation, the building of strong bones, heart function, and to assist in nerve impulse transmission. These minerals are split into two main groups and must be consumed in our diets. They are the five major minerals (calcium, phosphorous, potassium, sodium, and magnesium) and some trace minerals or elements (sulphur, iron, chlorine, cobalt, copper, zinc, manganese, molybdenum, iodine, and selenium). This list does not include chloride (chlorine), which is considered part of the compound sodium chloride (salt). The trace mineral sulphur is included, but can only be accessed in amino acids, and not in its elemental form. Fluoride (fluorine) is not included, as it is assessed differently, considered a fortification under the remit of licensed medicines or products. However, all three are valuable for human health, with only sodium chloride and sulphur compounds considered essential. Three other minerals that have shown measurable responses to variations in dietary intakes but have a paucity of data to support their uses are boron, silicon, and vanadium. For these reasons, no Estimated Average Requirements (EARs, nutrient intake values that are approximated to meet the requirement of half the healthy individuals in a group) need determining for these latter elements.[19]

Others

There are also some conditionally essential nutrients that can be made in the human body, but under certain circumstances, particularly if the system is under duress, may need to be consumed in the diet, thereby adding to our own self-manufactured quantities.

In addition, we need insoluble dietary fibre to help provide bowel bulk. This is considered non-essential as it contains no nutrient value. However, it does play a major role in our digestive health, and therefore consumption is of great value to us. Foods that have little, or no nutrient value are sometimes referred to as those containing "empty calories".

Supplements themselves are not a substitute for a good balanced diet, nevertheless, are sometimes necessary to ensure we get enough of the essential nutrients we need to maintain or improve our health, and to fill in any gaps in our diets.[20]

It is worth remembering that foods will often have varied nutrient content — but most fruits and vegetables, for example, contain high levels of vitamin C, which is essential for plant growth itself, and is an essential micronutrient and vital antioxidant for humans — indispensable for normal immune system function.[21] There are myriad nutrient combinations available in the animal and plant kingdoms. Often, the constituent parts in our diets work in synergy with others, the combined effects seemingly greater than the sum of their parts — a famous quote attributed to Aristotle, the famous philosopher from Ancient Greece — but this may hide the truth somewhat, in that complex systems are hard to elucidate, and as such seem mysterious until well understood, often through research. Studies add to our knowledge base, but absolute certainty as to how nutrients all work together, in combination, is hard to fully understand, and ongoing research is a constant requirement for improving our comprehension. An example of a complicated interaction between two different aspects of nutrition is one illuminated by the Pemba study. This showed that iron supplementation could have detrimental effects on gastrointestinal structural integrity. Consequently, the gut microbe balance could be altered in some individuals, with complex and unintended adverse immune system related effects, particularly in Malaria endemic areas.[22] Another example is the reciprocal relationship between copper and zinc absorption, one inhibiting the other. This is the reason we use words like, "may", "could", and "might" with reference to maintaining a healthy human profile. For the same reason, we try to avoid absolutes, such as the words "does" and "will", as so much new information is becoming available through ongoing research, and so much uncertainty exists in all complex systems.

Recommended Daily Intakes

As there are figures for suggested daily consumptions in this book, particularly for vitamins and minerals, I would like to describe the commonly used measures for nutritional recommendations, as they often differ historically, and from country to country. The Dietary Reference Intake (DRI) was first introduced in 1997 to embellish the existing guidelines known as Recommended Dietary Allowances (RDAs). The Dietary Reference Intakes (DRI values) differ from those used in nutrition labelling on food and dietary supplement products in the US and Canada. These Reference Daily Intakes (RDIs) and Daily Values (%DV) were based on outdated RDAs from 1968, but these were subsequently updated in 2016.[23] The DRIs provide several different types of reference values. The following information is taken from "A Consumer's Guide to the DRIs (Dietary Reference Intakes)".[24]

- Estimated Average Requirements (EARs): expected to satisfy the needs of 50% of the people in that age group based on a review of the available scientific literature.
- Recommended Dietary Allowances (RDAs): the daily dietary intake level of a nutrient considered sufficient by the Food and Nutrition Board of the Institute of Medicine to meet the requirements of 97.5% of healthy individuals in each life-stage and sex group.

This definition implies that the intake level would cause a harmful nutrient deficiency in just 2.5% of individuals. It is calculated based upon the EAR and is usually approximately 20% higher than the EAR itself.
- Adequate Intakes (AIs): these are used where no RDA has been established, but the amount is believed to be adequate for everyone in a particular demographic group.
- Tolerable upper intake levels (ULs): these upper limits are intended to caution against excessive intake of nutrients. This is the highest level of daily nutrient consumption, which is considered safe for, and cause no side effects in, 97.5% of healthy individuals in each life-stage and sex group. The European Food Safety Authority (EFSA) has also established ULs, which do not always agree with US ULs.[25]
- Acceptable Macronutrient Distribution Ranges (AMDRs): ranges of intakes specified as a percentage of total energy intake. Used for sources of energy, such as fats and carbohydrates.

All measures may be quoted in this book, but the reader will see RDAs, AIs, and ULs most frequently, and at the end of each relevant entry.

Pregnancy and Lactation

Good nutrition is vital during pregnancy and lactation, as mothers need to maintain their own physiological processes, whilst also supporting foetal development. Placental and foetal growth is most vulnerable to the mother's nutritional status during the peri-implantation period (early stages of development) and the first trimester of gestation (the rapid phase of placental development). It is known that either maternal undernutrition or overnutrition throughout the whole pregnancy term can impede foetal growth.[26] It follows that there is a requirement for increased daily intakes of micronutrients of the right kinds and in the correct quantities, and even in industrialised countries there are risks of inadequate amounts being consumed. This particularly applies to docosahexaenoic acid (DHA), an omega-3 fatty acid, the minerals iron, iodine, calcium, and vitamins B9 (Folic acid or folate), vitamin C, and vitamin D. During pregnancy both maternal tissues and foetal growth require increased protein consumption, particularly in the third trimester. Again, we do not need to consume more than is necessary, as excessive protein consumption can be detrimental to both the mother and the developing foetus.[27] The quality of fat is important, with DHA intake of utmost importance for foetal brain, retinal development, and psychomotor neurodevelopment in the first few months of life.[28] Insufficient folic acid during pregnancy has been linked to increased risks of neural tube defects — this is the reason some countries, including the US, Canada, South Africa, Chile, and Costa Rica have initiated fortification programs. These were made mandatory in the US and Canada back in 1998.[29] As recently as July 2021, New Zealand mandated fortification with folic acid, and following a 2019 consultation, the UK Government announced on September 20th, 2021, that it would introduce the mandatory fortification of non-wholemeal wheat flour with folic acid.[30]

The first 1,000 days of life for a child are believed to represent a particularly important period — this is roughly the time between conception and a child`s second birthday. During this period optimal maternal nutrition is essential for infant growth, also reducing the risks of developing some adult diseases later in life. Breast milk, which contains nutrients and bioactive factors needed for infant health and development, is considered the gold standard, and is recommended by the World Cancer Research Fund as an important factor for the prevention of cancer in the lactating mother too.[31]

What to Avoid in Pregnancy?

Whilst vitamin A is a crucial micronutrient for both expectant women and the foetus, taking vitamin A supplements, or consuming foods containing high levels of retinol (vitamin A1), a derivative of vitamin A — only found in animal-sourced foods, including oily fish, cheese and butter, eggs, and liver can be dangerous. This is because vitamin A can exert teratogenic effects; those effects, which might disturb the development of the embryo or foetus, particularly in the first 60 days following conception.[32] Cheese, milk, and other dairy products should be pasteurised, as unpasteurised foods may contain listeria — a bacteria that can cause a damaging infection, known as listeriosis. Meats and poultry should be well-cooked, as they may contain parasites that could cause the disease toxoplasmosis. Game can retain lead shot, so should be avoided, or at least checked very carefully. Eggs should be cooked well, or have been processed correctly, to kill off any salmonella bacteria, and some fish can contain high levels of mercury, a toxin, often found in concentrated forms in tuna, swordfish, and some shellfish. As a precaution, these are best avoided. Some advice also relates to moderation of alcohol and reducing caffeine intake, avoiding consumption of liquorice root, rationing herbal teas, as well as washing all fruit and vegetables to clean off soil deposits.

Microbiome & Immunity

Many vitamins and minerals are essential for supporting the immune system, which protects us from infection. Whilst maintaining good health is certainly dependent upon good nutrition, it may also be reliant upon having a well constituted human microbiome.[33] The collective term microbiome is used to represent the genomes (genetic material) of microorganisms or microbiota that reside inside us. A large number are found in the human gut, and there are many microorganisms that colonise our skin, most of which are beneficial or harmless to us. There are an estimated 20,000-25,000, maybe more, human protein-coding genes, and these microbes add well over another additional 100,000 genes, outnumbering our own genes by a factor of between five and ten. They work symbiotically with us, to provide beneficial traits that humans did not need to evolve by themselves; a great deal of evolutionary energy was saved in this manner.[34] There is also a link between specific blood types and the different bacterial strains that make up the microbiome, which like to use specific blood type antigens as preferred food sources. The immune system and digestive systems retain a memory, a type of favouritism, for foods that our ancestors used to eat. This means different blood groups, whether O, A, B, or AB, have differently evolved microbiota and consequently different predilections for food types. For example, blood type O individuals are considered hunter-gatherers and are good at digesting protein, but are often gluten intolerant, whereas blood type A individuals prefer an agrarian diet containing plant proteins and carbohydrates, and they are consequently better adapted to digest these foods.[35] Concerning blood groups, an article from China examining 2,173 patients with COVID-19, (the infectious disease responsible for the ongoing pandemic and caused by the most recently discovered coronavirus) confirmed by the SARS-CoV-2 test in three hospitals in Wuhan and Shenzhen, found an association between blood group type and the risks of contracting COVID-19. The results showed blood group A individuals were at higher risk of acquiring COVID-19, when compared with non-A blood groups, and blood group O individuals were at lower risk of acquiring the infection ,when compared with non-O blood groups. The article was at pains to emphasise the early nature of the study and its limitations, but concluded that "it should encourage further investigation of the relationship between the ABO blood groups and COVID-19 susceptibility".[36] According to mathematicians, Christian Yates and colleagues, all the COVID-19 in the world could comfortably fit into a coke tin, with room to spare.[37] The findings on blood groups could fit in with other reported research on blood types and predictions for possible individual susceptibility to certain diseases. Blood type O individuals may have a lower risk of heart disease, but higher risks of stomach ulcers, and blood type A people may have higher risks of acquiring microbial infections.[38]

Between the years of 2000 and 2001, I personally suffered from the symptoms of chronic fatigue syndrome (CFS). It is also known as "ME", which stands for myalgic encephalomyelitis, and many people refer to the condition as "CFS/ME". Other names include Post-Viral Fatigue Syndrome or "PVFS" and Chronic Fatigue Immune Dysfunction Syndrome or "CFIDS". NHS UK describes the illness as a long-term illness, with a wide range of symptoms, the most common of which is extreme tiredness. My symptoms lasted for nearly a year, so maybe I was lucky, as so many people live with this condition for many years, if not most of their lives. I wanted to share my experience with the reader, as I thought it might help others to try and fathom out the possible causes of their own illness. My condition appeared, after considerable reflection, to be related to my own gut microbiota balance, or imbalance. The main symptom that I experienced was, indeed, extreme tiredness and often prolonged periods of fatigue. At that time, I could have slept, and often did, for many hours a day without ever feeling truly refreshed. My own personal salvation came from some advice given to me by a patient, who suggested that I should rebalance my gut. I thought about this and together with my own doctor we reappraised my medical history. During the consultation I recalled a trip abroad earlier in the year, when I acquired a stomach infection, and subsequently relayed the recollection to my doctor that I had felt mildly poisoned ever since that holiday, and particularly unwell following subsequent antibiotic treatment. My GP thought it may have been caused by a bacterial or viral infection of some sort. I wondered if the wide-spectrum antibiotics might well have been, at the very least, a partial cause of the ensuing condition. It is now known that the abnormal presence of pathogenic or toxigenic microorganisms in the intestine may lead in certain circumstances to gastrointestinal infection, and that reducing the numbers of specific pathogenic organisms in these ecosystems can be beneficial for the overall physiology. Moreover, the presence of pathogens and/or toxinogenic microorganisms in the gastrointestinal tract is also thought to be a risk factor for infections themselves. Therefore, reducing the numbers of these microorganisms, and the toxins they produce, can be potentially important for good overall gut function.[39] So, a bit of chicken and egg there! There are now many reports of pathogens and/or toxigenic microorganisms in the gastrointestinal tract, which proliferate following antibiotic treatment, and can cause systemic problems. Antimicrobial treatment is known to disrupt the microbiome — consisting of about 10-100 trillion symbiotic microbial cells within the human gut of every person, and just a single antibiotic dose can cause unforeseen effects by killing many of these beneficial bacteria. Antibiotics alter the microbiome composition, which can result in an increased risk of disease, secondary infections, allergies, and obesity. Also, it is known that the spread of drug resistant pathogens can be promoted within the general environment by antibiotic overuse.[40] Clinical resistance to antimicrobials was, believe it or not, first seen and reported upon four years before the discovery of penicillin by Alexander Fleming in 1928. The antimicrobial agent concerned was called Salvarsan.[41] The first sign of antibiotic resistance to penicillin, itself, became apparent fairly soon after its discovery. In 1940, Abraham and Chain reported an enzyme, a penicillinase, present in an E. coli bacteria strain that could inactivate the relatively recently discovered penicillin.[42]

The human microbiome consists of mainly bacteria, but also archaea (single-celled microorganisms, which are comparable to bacteria and are at least 2.7 billion years old), fungi, protists, (another ancient group of single-celled organisms), and many viruses. Mounting evidence shows there may be a link between the human microbiome and the influence this may have on the function of the gut and wider immune system.[43] By extension, the thought was by rebalancing my own gut microbiome, this could have a beneficial impact? My own personal treatment consisted of taking just three concentrated doses of Lactobacillus Acidophilus, an important bacterium found in the human intestines, for around a two-week period. Following this, I felt at least a ninety per cent improvement, with only a temporary relapse, or a shadow of the symptoms returning a few weeks later after contracting the common cold (viral). I have not had the same symptoms of fatigue since, and this treatment occurred nearly 20 years ago. As an osteopath, I recognise that disruptions to the structure can also put strains on the musculo-skeletal and nervous systems. These will often predispose to other problems, such as increased infection risk, gut imbalance, and other visceral (relating to the organs) problems, through complex interactions and reflexes. This is the reason, quite often, we label complex conditions, often calling them syndromes, but this by extension can label the patient. This can cause confusion and consequently does not elucidate all the possible causes, but simply lists a group of symptoms, which consistently occur together, or refers to a condition that is characterised by a set of associated symptoms. This is also the case with "CFS/ME" syndrome, which is believed to affect more than 250,000 people across the UK. But in no way could I say that precisely the same treatment I received, and derived benefit from, would help someone else — as disease description and symptom patterns are highly individualised and complex in their nature. The hope is that this can help others consider more of the possibilities that can be appraised and might help to facilitate health improvement in those individuals. A fellow osteopath, Dr Raymond Perrin, has delved into various structural links and has arrived at the firm conclusion that "ME" is a structural disorder with definite diagnosable physical signs — the gut is part of our structure of course.[44]

We could all consider and explore more holistic thought processes, by considering as many factors as possible in our approach for supporting good health. I think holism could be defined in this fashion; trying to look at as many components that are considered relevant and present in complex systems, affected by many, often, inter-related factors. If we can then be specific in our solutions, with targeted responses, which does not mean do everything, in many cases this can allow natural balance to be restored. Holistic thought considers and appraises many elements but can be specific in action. Later in the book I will discuss prebiotics and probiotics, elements that help the microbiome stay balanced, which are used in food supplements, and are found, often together, in many food types; these combinations are referred to as synbiotics, and these are thought to be important for gastrointestinal function.

The relationship between structure and function is intrinsic to all and represents an important osteopathic principle. This inextricable link is often phrased in the following manner- "structure governing function". However, those functions that confer survivability in the environment, need to evolve structures to fulfil them over time. So, this means, in a way, function also governs structure — effectively a bidirectional relationship exists. The following section talks about the beneficial incorporation of some unusual genetic material, which has helped humans to thrive and prosper.

Viruses & Their Role in the Human Microbiome

Viruses interact with the genetic material in most cells, the building blocks of all living things. This includes the trillions that are present and stable in the human microbiome. Some of these viruses can even be found in the bloodstream, previously thought to be a sterile environment. There is a huge diversity of viruses found in humans, many of which infect bacteria, and are known as bacteriophages — literally meaning bacteria eaters. In fact, some viruses can provide evolutionary advantages to certain bacteria, but others can cause an imbalance between the natural organisms residing in a person's natural microflora, especially in the gut, and are thought to contribute to a range of illnesses, such as Crohn's disease.[45]

Such is our intrinsic and long-standing relationship with viruses that the human genome itself contains roughly 100,000 pieces of viral DNA, or to put it another way, the pieces make up around 8 percent of the total human genome.[46] This is about four times more than the Neanderthal-genetic material that modern non-African humans have inherited. The human genome was 99% mapped by 2003, thanks to the Human Genome Project, with nearly all 3.2 billion base pairs sequenced; part of around 30,000 human genes, or certainly more than 25,000.[47] One piece of our DNA controls production of a retroviral envelope protein called "Hemo", which is believed to have entered our ancestors' genomes around 100 million years ago, and seems to be important in regulating human pregnancy. Retroviruses, as a group, may have become integrated into the DNA of two major lineages of ray-finned fish as long ago as 450 million years, probably before the advent of any jawed vertebrate hosts. These probably arose in the Late Silurian Period, more than 416 million years ago.[48]

Hierarchy of Evidence

Depending on which source one uses, most people have seen the hierarchy shown below (Fig 5).

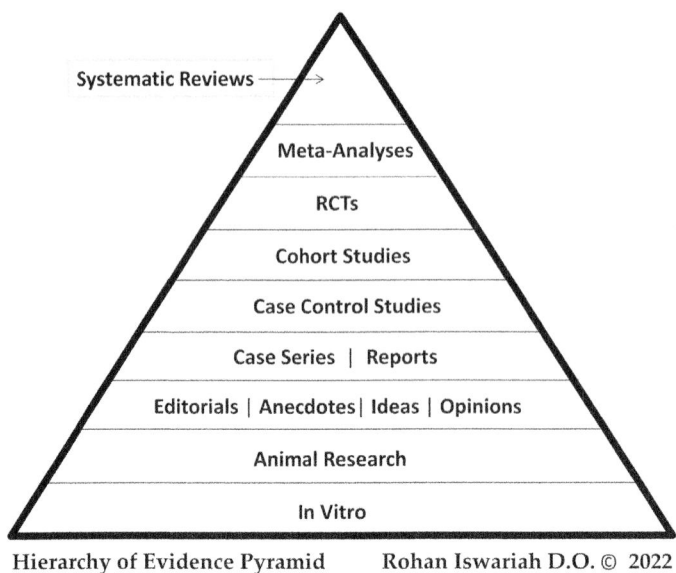

Hierarchy of Evidence Pyramid   Rohan Iswariah D.O. © 2022

This concerns the power of research and evidence, and how much credence to attach to evidence imparted on a variety of subjects, including nutritional advice. It is based upon its perceived reliability. This list describes in order from the strongest first, descending to the lowest valued evidence at the base of the pyramid. A pictorial representation, called a pyramid of hierarchy, as shown above, which many believe could be a slightly flawed valuation. Randomised Controlled Trials (RCTs) tend to measure one intervention or variable against controls, and as most systems are complex, they are not necessarily best, or solely, suited to RCTs. Therefore, the addition of satisfaction studies (which relate to individual experience), surveys, and other observational tools can be useful additions to the information afforded by RCTs themselves. There can be manifold possible errors in meta-analyses too. Overall, the model shown represents a good system, which can be embellished by anecdotal experience and empirical information, as garnered through our senses.

- Systematic reviews: a summary of all the studies addressing a specific question.
- Meta-analyses: data is taken from individual studies and can be united quantitatively and re-analysed.
- Randomised controlled double-blind studies or trials (RCTs): studies where people are allocated at random to receive one of several clinical interventions, which are then compared.
- Cohort studies: over time, the sampling of a group of people who share defining characteristics that are therefore similar.
- Case-control studies: these are non-experimental comparisons.
- Case series and reports: these can be extremely detailed but are also non-experimental in nature.
- Editorials, ideas, and opinions: I could include anecdotal evidence here — relying heavily or entirely upon personal testimony, but not without value.
- Animal research.
- In-vitro ("test tube") research: literally meaning "in glass". Compounds or constituents of an organism are studied outside of their usual biological milieu.

Philosophy of Health

We need to remember that a good philosophy for staying healthy should be based primarily around a healthy lifestyle, allied with the correct advice. NHS UK [49] suggests the following: giving up smoking, staying active, managing weight, eating more fibre, cutting down on saturated fat, eating at least five portions of a variety of fruit and vegetables a day, eating fish at least twice a week, drinking less alcohol and cutting down on salt to maintain a healthy blood pressure. High salt levels are directly correlated with certain health problems; extra water becomes stored, because of the presence of salt, causing an increased blood pressure, which can directly and detrimentally affect the heart, arteries, kidneys, and brain. Additionally, some diuretic medications, which patients are prescribed, are rendered less affective by excessive salt consumption. It is thought that nearly 80% of the salt we eat every day is "hidden" in processed foods, and it is generally considered advisable to keep abreast of all available health information by reading labels carefully and understanding how amounts can fit in with a healthy personal lifestyle. Too much sugar can also cause health problems, and according to NHS UK research, children are consuming twice as much sugar as they need, of which half of the intake is from unhealthy snacks and sugary drinks.[50] Adults also consume far too much sugar, which is often found in the highest amounts in a wide range of foods, such as: fizzy drinks and fruit juices, breakfast cereals and yoghurt, sweets, chocolate and ice-cream, cakes and buns, pastries and biscuits, sauces, condiments and salad dressings, bread (which is not usually thought of as a sweet food), cereal and nutrition bars (some have added sugar), jams and jellies, and many other processed foods. This is a long list but is by no means exhaustive, so we really need to look carefully at labels, as lots of these foods are often mistakenly assumed to be healthy. A special issue of the journal "Public Health Nutrition" showed that UK families bought more ultra-processed food than others in Europe, amounting to around 50.7% of our diets. Germany came second, followed by Ireland. These figures came from national surveys and demonstrated trends that were acknowledged not to be completely comparable, but they do represent "food for thought".[51] On occasions, we still need to fill in the gaps in our diets with supplementation, so that a good balanced nutritional state can be maintained. The alphabetical list that follows is not exhaustive, but contains all the main vitamins and minerals, many herbs, and some of the most common ingredients used in food supplements and extracts.

A

Vitamin A

Vitamin A is a fat-soluble vitamin that includes retinol. It is found in foods from animal sources and carotenoids, the yellow-orange pigments mainly derived from plants such as carrots, tomatoes, corn, and some fungi. Some studies show that increased retinol and carotene absorption can be achieved by increasing the level of fat consumed in the diet, particularly in a low-fat diet scenario. Pairing any of the fat-soluble vitamins with fat maximises absorption, but where possible the fat source should be a largely unsaturated one, such as: peanut and sesame oil, other nuts, seeds, olives or olive oil, and avocados.

Vitamin A is essential for normal growth and development, immune function, and vision. Immune function depends on cell differentiation and proliferation in response to immune stimuli, and retinoic acids or retinoids are important for the maintenance of circulating natural killer cells that protect against viruses and help anti-tumour activity.[52] Consequently, it is needed in higher amounts during times of infection, as it plays such an important role in T-cell (a type of lymphocyte, which comes from the thymus gland) production. Vision is reliant upon vitamin A-based photoreceptor proteins known as opsins, which have been used for billions of years to sense light in vision, or the equivalent of vision within the animal kingdom.[53] Vitamin A also helps to maintain healthy skin, teeth, bones, and mucous membranes.

No single event can be called the discovery of vitamin A, but an understanding of its nature arose from incremental processes over a period of around 130 years. In 1816, François Magendie found corneal ulcers and higher mortality rates in dogs deprived of certain nutrition, which was comparable with the clinical findings in poorly fed, abandoned infants in Paris, France, in the same time frame. In the mid-to-late 1800s Nicolai Lunin, a Russian doctor, conducted an experiment with two groups of mice. He found those fed with milk fared much better than the other group fed with a combination of proteins, fats, carbohydrates, and minerals consistent with the proportions found in cow`s milk. He concluded that there was an unknown substance in milk, essential to nutrition, which he called "inorganic salts" — now known as vitamin A. Various scientists, including Carl Socin, Frederick Gowland, Wilhelm Stepp, Elmer McCollum and Marguerite Davis, Thomas Osbourne and Lafayette Mendel advanced our knowledge until Paul Karrer described the actual chemical structure of vitamin A in 1932.[54] [55]

It is now estimated that nearly one-third of children under the age of five, worldwide, are vitamin A deficient.[56] The recommended daily allowance (RDA) is around 800 mcg per day, but it must be remembered that it is important not to exceed 3,000 mcg, as vitamin A has a defined therapeutic window and excesses need to be avoided, especially during pregnancy. Vitamin A enters the nervous system with greater ease than most other vitamins due to its fat-solubility, and toxic levels can accumulate with slow disposal rates. Animal liver is very high in vitamin A, as this is where it is stored. It is advised to avoid eating too many liver or animal products containing the preformed vitamin A (retinol) during pregnancy. Eating vegetables containing carotenoids is a useful way to obtain vitamin A. Daily requirements, adequate intakes, and upper limits are shown below.[57]

Recommended Dietary Allowances (RDAs)

- AI (Adequate Intake) in infants 0-6 months: 400 mcg of retinol activity equivalents (RAE) per day based upon average milk intake of 0.78 litres per day
- AI in infants 7-12 months: 500 mcg RAE per day
- Recommended Daily Allowance (RDA) 1-3 years: 300 mcg RAE per day
- RDA 4-8 years: 400 mcg RAE per day
- RDA for boys 9-13 years: 600 mcg RAE per day
- RDA for boys 14-18 years: 900 mcg RAE per day
- RDA for girls 9-13 years: 600 mcg RAE per day
- RDA for girls 14-18 years: 700 mcg RAE per day
- RDA for men 19-70 plus years: 900 mcg RAE per day
- RDA for women 19-70 plus years: 700 mcg RAE per day
- RDA for pregnancy 14-18 years: 750 mcg RAE per day
- RDA for pregnancy 19-30 years: 770 mcg RAE per day
- RDA for pregnancy 31-50 years: 770 mcg RAE per day
- RDA for lactation 14-18 years: 1,200 mcg RAE per day
- RDA for lactation 19-30 years: 1,300 mcg RAE per day
- RDA for lactation 31-50 years: 1,300 mcg RAE per day

Tolerable upper limits vary according to age and are shown below.

Upper limits (ULs)

- 0-12 months: 600 mcg per day of preformed vitamin A
- 1-3 years: 600 mcg per day of preformed vitamin A
- 4-8 years: 900 mcg per day of preformed vitamin A
- 9-13 years: 1,700 mcg per day of preformed vitamin A
- For boys 14-18 years: 2,800 mcg per day of preformed vitamin A
- For women 14-18 years: 2,800 mcg per day of preformed vitamin A
- For men over 19 years: 3,000 mcg per day of preformed vitamin A

- For women 19 years and upwards: 3,000 mcg per day of preformed vitamin A
- For women 14-18 years who are pregnant or lactating: 2,800 mcg per day of preformed vitamin A

Acai Berries -Euterpe Oleraceae

These berries are more accurately described as drupes, as they contain a single pit rather like an olive. The drupes are the fruits of the acai palm, believed to be endowed with medicinal properties by the indigenous peoples of the Brazilian rainforest. The acai is just one of several thousand rainforest fruits native to various countries, including Brazil and Peru, mainly growing in swamps and on floodplains. The word "acai", in the native tongue of peoples from tropical Central and South America, translates as the "fruit that cries". The fruits are considered the "source of life" as they contain high fibre levels, vitamins A and C, iron, calcium, omega fatty acids (3,6, and 9), proteins, and anthocyanins. They have shown significantly high antioxidant capacity in-vitro, and therefore may have additional health benefits. Anti-inflammatory and immune functions were investigated in a 2006 study, where the acai was found to be a potential, emphasis on the word potential, cyclooxygenase (COX-1 and COX-2) inhibitor.[58] The COX enzymes are known to produce prostaglandins. These are compounds that promote inflammation, pain, and fever, and therefore by inhibiting them to some extent a reduction in inflammation and pain can be achieved. There is no definitive evidence, based upon human studies, that support acai use for any specific health-related claims, and no peer-reviewed journals that can substantiate claims that acai alone can promote rapid weight loss. One preliminary study has suggested, however, that eating the fruit pulp might reduce sugar and cholesterol levels in already overweight people.[59]

Acerola Cherry -Malpighia emarginata

This bright red fruit or drupe contains approximately 50-100 times more vitamin C than that of either an orange or lemon.[60] Other familiar names for this fruit are the Barbados cherry, West Indian cherry, and wild crepe myrtle. It is also rich in vitamins A, B_1, B_2, and B_3, in addition to carotenoids and bioflavonoids. These all provide important nutritional value and may have antioxidant properties too.[61] Acerola is native to Central America, southern Mexico, and the Caribbean, and can also provide a high level of the trace element manganese, which we need in increasing amounts as we get older.[62]

African Mango -Irvingia gabonensis

The tree is also known as the wild mango. The nuts from the actual fruit of this tall African tree are rich in fats, proteins, and contain soluble fibre. The edible seeds are nutritious and consumed in large quantities in Africa. The spicy, earthy fruit also contains several minerals, and vitamin C.

Alfalfa -Medicago sativa

This perennial flowering plant, also known as Lucerne, has sprouting seeds containing vitamin C, some B vitamins, vitamin K, phosphorus, and zinc — also containing low levels of fat. It is an important fodder crop used to feed animals worldwide and is native to the warmer middle latitudes. People use the leaves, sprouts, and seeds to make medicine, but care needs to be taken with the raw unsprouted alfalfa seeds. These have toxic effects in primates, which includes humans of course. The raw seeds and sprouts contain the plant amino acid canavanine, which competes with arginine (a semi-essential or conditionally essential amino acid) that is important for protein building in humans. Most of the canavanine is converted into other amino acids during germination, therefore the sprouts contain much less canavanine than the unsprouted seeds, and consequently are safer.[63] The US National Institutes of Health also warn that alfalfa interacts with Warfarin based drugs in a major way, and the two should never be combined.[64]

Aloe Vera

This is a succulent plant native to Africa, which has been valued for thousands of years for its medicinal properties. Usage can be traced back 6,000 years to early Egypt where it was known as the "plant of immortality". Papyrus writings describe its anti-inflammatory and pain-relieving properties. Cleopatra was said to use it every day to keep her skin smooth and supple, and it was known as the "elixir of life" by the pharaohs. Around 3,000 BC, aloe vera starts appearing in Chinese and Sumerian writings, two of the five original writing systems, but only Chinese has survived into the modern age.[65] During the Greco-Roman era, aloe was thought to heal wounds and boils, to prevent hair loss, and alleviate skin conditions.[66] Aloe vera contains seventy-five potentially active constituents, including: vitamins, enzymes, minerals, sugars, lignin, saponins, salicylic acids, and amino acids.[67] However, there is evidence that adverse interactions are possible with some prescription drugs, particularly when Aloe vera is ingested in product form. Nevertheless, it is sometimes taken orally for conditions, including bowel diseases and fever, but most often the two substances from aloe vera (the clear gel and the yellow latex) are applied topically to the skin to treat burns, frostbite, psoriasis, and cold sores. There is some evidence that topical use of aloe products could be helpful in relieving the symptoms of psoriasis and some other rashes.[68]

Alpha-Linolenic Acid

This is an essential fatty acid, also known as ALA. Omega-3-ALA is found in English walnuts, chia seeds, flaxseed, and vegetable oils. Animals that feed on ALA-rich grasses are another important source of this omega-3 fatty acid. ALA and linolenic acid need to be acquired from dietary sources and are therefore considered essential for humans. Other long chain omega-3 oils, such as DHA (Docosahexaenoic acid) and EPA (Eicosapentaenoic acid), are not considered essential as they can be manufactured in the human body. The daily Adequate Intakes (AIs) for omega-3s are shown below. For infants, the AIs apply to total omega-3s. For ages 1 and upwards, the AIs apply just to ALA, because ALA is the only omega-3 that is essential.[69]

Adequate Intakes (AIs)

- 0-12 months 0.5 g as total omega-3s
- 1-3 years 0.7 g
- 4-8 years 0.9 g
- 9-13 years male: 1.2 g female 1.0 g
- 14-18 years male: 1.6 g female 1.1 g
- Men 1.6 g
- Women 1.1 g
- Pregnant teens and women 1.4 g
- Breastfeeding teens and women 1.3 g

Alpha-Lipoic-Acid

This acronym, ALA, is not to be confused with the previous entry. This acid is not an omega-3 essential fatty acid. However, it is an important compound required for aerobic metabolism. It is commonly found in mitochondria (the powerhouses within cells) and is necessary for several different enzymatic functions. It is also considered a powerful antioxidant that is involved, as a cofactor, in several important enzyme systems. Data shows that bioavailability can be poor due to its breakdown in the liver. ALA is found in many vegetables, including spinach, broccoli, Brussels sprouts, tomatoes, rice bran, meats, liver, and kidneys. It can be synthesised in mitochondria using compounds, which include the amino acid cysteine.[70]

Apple Cider Vinegar

Apple cider vinegar is made by fermenting the slurry of pulp and juice using yeast, and then reducing the alcohol into vinegar by using acetic acid-forming bacteria. Some papers have recorded health benefits, including a reduction in glucose response to carbohydrate loading in both healthy adults and individuals with diabetes. There is also some evidence that vinegar ingestion increases short-term satiety or satisfaction of hunger pangs.[71] Other than these weak findings, there are no proven benefits for skin conditions or weight loss. Uses date back to nearly 3,300 BC, but are mostly anecdotal, and Samurai warriors, more recently, are thought to have used apple cider vinegar as an invigorating tonic to both increase strength and power. A lack of any good current data means that safety cannot be assessed and therefore ingestion is not recommended in pregnant and breastfeeding women.[72]

Arnica- Arnica Montana

Arnica is an aromatic perennial belonging to the sunflower family. The flowers are golden-yellow and contain a lactone known as helenalin. This is considered the active ingredient, which is used in anti-inflammatory creams and gels. Helenalin suppresses cytokine formation, one of the pro-inflammatory substances widely distributed and circulating in the human body. However, helenalin is toxic if consumed in large amounts. Arnica likes to grow in alpine settings throughout Europe, although these days it is becoming rarer and less widely distributed due to wild foraging. Traditionally, Arnica was used as a folk medicine for bruising, to alleviate pain, help with acne, sore throats, chapped lips, and insect bites. Some research shows that using an arnica gel cream twice daily for a period of three weeks can reduce pain and stiffness, as well as helping with movement of the hands and knees, for sufferers of osteoarthritis.[73] Other research has shown that Arnica is probably at least as good as ibuprofen in improving function and reducing pain in osteoarthritis of the hands.[74] A lot of people believe arnica use stems from the 16th century, when it was widely used in Germany for treating bruising and inflammation. Goethe, the famous writer, statesman and scientist, known as the Shakespeare of Germany, was thought to have regularly brewed tea using this herb as part of a recovery program following a heart attack; his health improved – this was attributed in part to Arnica.[75] Nowadays it is most often used in topical form around the world, including the US.

Artichoke- Cynara cardunculus var scolymus

The globe artichoke has buds that are edible and contain the bitter flavoured lactone cynaropicrin. Artichoke is related to the thistle, part of the sunflower family, and has long been cultivated as a food. Its origins go back more than 2,000 years to ancient Greece. The name was originally derived from a Ligurian word cocali, meaning pine cone, which its shape sort of resembles.[76] Liguria is a region of north-western Italy, the capital is Genoa, and artichokes are still one of the most common and popular vegetables in the whole of Italy today. The health benefits of cynaropicrin are well documented; the most outstanding of which is the anti-Hepatitis C viral properties, which could help develop preventive therapies/measures against hepatitis C in the future. Cynaropicrin can also suppress hyperlipidaemia (raised serum cholesterol levels), has potent antioxidant effects, and inhibits some inflammatory mediators.[77]

Ashwagandha- Withania somnifera

The powdered root of this plant, also known as Indian ginseng, is a member of the nightshade family that has been used in Indian Ayurvedic medicine as a potent regenerative tonic for centuries. Recent research shows it may have multiple effects, which include anti-stress, neuroprotective, antitumour, anti-arthritic, analgesic, and anti-inflammatory properties.[78] Following appraisal of all the available research, "Medline plus" concluded that taking a specific ashwagandha root extract appeared to improve the symptoms of stress, but also concluded that there was insufficient evidence to rate effectiveness for a host of other medical conditions. However, by taking a specific ashwagandha extract (Strelaxin 400 mg) three times daily for one month, this could reduce levels of fat and sugars. Other research showed that taking ashwagandha could reduce symptoms of anxiety — an extract taken for 8 weeks might improve brain function in people having treatment for bipolar disorder (a mental health condition causing extreme mood swings). There is also some evidence to show its cholesterol-lowering effects in patients with high cholesterol, and that taking ashwagandha could help people with a mild form of underactive thyroid. Ashwagandha is believed to contain chemicals that might help calm the brain, reduce inflammation, and alter the immune system.[79]

Astragalus- Astragalus membranaceus & Astragalus mongholicus

The root of the astragalus plant has been used for centuries in Chinese medicine, often allied with other popular herbs such as ginseng, dong quai, and liquorice. Two of the species commonly used in supplements are Astragalus membranaceus and

Astragalus mongholicus, but over 3,000 species of this small shrub or herb are known to exist. Common names include milkvetch, goat`s-thorn, and locoweed. Traditional medicinal uses included treatment for diarrhoea, fatigue, anorexia, upper respiratory infections, heart disease, hepatitis, fibromyalgia (a condition that causes widespread pain and is often called fibromyalgia syndrome), and some adjunctive uses for cancer therapy. Astragalus benefits for these health conditions have not been backed up by any high-quality studies to date, although, some weak evidence for astragalus helping heart function in some patients with a viral infection of the heart was uncovered in a 2013 research review.[80] Another more recent review and article from 2020 looking into the active compounds in astragalus (A. membranaceus) found that astragalus polysaccharide (APS) was the most important. This water-soluble compound with bioactive effects might offer great advantages for the treatment of diabetes mellitus and its complications (a condition causing high blood glucose levels with the sugars eventually excreted in the urine). As a natural drug, it was considered suitable for long-term use in patients with this chronic disease, but it was still deemed important to elucidate the actual mechanism of action in diabetes mellitus.[81]

Astaxanthin

This compound gives some fish a pink hue. It is a naturally occurring carotenoid found in algae, shrimp, lobster, crab, and salmon that remains under preliminary research. EFSA concluded in February 2020 that an intake of 8 mg of ATX per day from food supplements was safe for adults.[82]

Avocado- Persea Americana

The Avocado is a tree thought to have originated from Mexico but might well have been more widespread. The tree produces fruit, a large berry, with a flavour often described as rich and mellow with a buttery consistency. The fruit of the avocado tree contains several beneficial nutrients, including omega-6 and omega-9 fatty acids, vitamins B, C, E, and K, potassium, copper, and contains good fibre content too. The leaves are considered harmful to many animals and the fruit is poisonous to some birds. The toxic compound is persin, a fungicide that is mainly found in the leaves, with relatively low concentrations in the ripe pulp of the avocado fruit itself. It is generally considered harmless to humans.[83]

Ayurveda and herbs

Ayurveda or Ayurvedic medicine is the traditional medicinal system used for thousands of years across the Indian subcontinent. A wide range of remedies based upon herbs and plant compounds, minerals, and metal substances are thought to have many health benefits. The remedies are generally used as combinations of plants, herbs, and minerals, and rarely in isolation. The philosophy of Indian medicine also embraces diet, exercise, and lifestyle, thus underpinning an holistic approach. There are a few trials and studies that demonstrate benefits using modern evidence-based criteria. One 2013 study into knee osteoarthritis lasting 6 months concluded that Ayurvedic formulations, which contained extracts of Tinospora cordifolia (Guduchi stem), Zingiber officinale (Ginger root), Emblica officinalis (Amalaki fruit), and Boswellia serrata (Boswellia) significantly reduced knee pain and improved knee function in osteoarthritis sufferers. These benefits were equivalent to the group randomly assigned to glucosamine and celecoxib (a non-steroidal anti-inflammatory drug) treatment.[84] A pilot study in 2011 comparing classical Ayurveda and methotrexate treatment (a type of medicine used as an immunosuppressant) — demonstrated equal benefits; with the Ayurvedic group experiencing fewer adverse side-effects than the methotrexate group.[85] Another review found the use of some herbal mixtures was associated with significant glucose-lowering effects, but questioned the small sample sizes used in several of the appraised studies.[86] Small studies into turmeric in 2005 and 2006 thought that its active ingredient curcumin could be helpful for ulcerative colitis sufferers. A more recent 2012 preclinical study in animals showed that curcumin was effective in preventing or ameliorating ulcerative colitis, also reducing inflammation.[87] We now know that piperine, a compound found in black pepper, can increase the bioavailability of curcumin, the active ingredient sourced from turmeric roots. Both piperine and curcumin are often found together in supplements for this reason. However, some Ayurvedic combinations contain metals, minerals, and gems. Metal content, particularly, is considered potentially quite harmful, according to the US Food and Drug Administration.[88]

B

Vitamin B1

Vitamin B1, also known as thiamine or thiamin, is a water-soluble vitamin and therefore excreted in the urine on a daily basis. We have low stores that need constant replenishing — consequently, we need to consume sufficient quantities in our diets where possible. Found in whole grains, legumes, fish, and meats (especially pork and duck), it is easily lost during food processing. Thiamin is destroyed with high heat cooking, such as boiling. As it is water-soluble it tends to leach out during these cooking methods, also during the canning and preserving processes too. It plays a vital role in nerve, muscle, and heart function, and is essential for energy production using glucose. Thiamine deficiency can cause the medical condition beriberi, which has two forms, wet and dry beriberi. The word `beriberi` is thought to have originated from the Singhalese (Sri Lankan, originally Ceylonese) language and means either `weak` or `I cannot`, which is repeated for emphasis. This derivation could be due to the higher prevalence of the disease in Southeast Asia, as opposed to Europe where it has been largely eradicated. Many scientists have studied vitamin B1, but it was the Polish-American scientist, Casimir Funk, who first isolated it from brown rice in 1912, and was attributed with the discovery. Initially it was described as the `anti-beriberi factor`, and subsequently the word vitamin was used, which is derived from the Latin `vita` (meaning life) and `amine` (as vitamins were thought to contain amino acids — a group of nitrogen-containing organic molecules). He also postulated the existence of a number of other compounds or `vitamines`, which might have been necessary for disease prevention.[89] Wet beriberi affects the cardiovascular system and dry beriberi tends to affect the nervous system. Wet beriberi symptoms, include increased heart rate, shortness of breath, and swelling of the lower legs. Dry beriberi sufferers can experience difficulty in walking, loss of feeling in the hands and/or feet, paralysis of the lower legs, mental confusion, speech difficulty, pain, and/or vomiting.[90] EFSA suggests the maximum daily intake from all thiamine sources, including supplements, should not exceed 100 mg per day.[91] No upper limits have been published though, as excess thiamine is excreted in the urine. RDAs for vitamin B1 are shown below.[92]

Recommended Dietary Allowances (RDAs)

- 0-6 months: male 0.2 mg: female 0.2 mg, also AI
- 7-12 months: male 0.3 mg: female 0.3 mg, also AI
- 1-3 years: male 0.5 mg: female 0.5 mg
- 4-8 years: male 0.6 mg: female 0.6 mg
- 9-13 years: male 0.9 mg: female 0.9 mg
- 14-18 years: male 1.2 mg: female 1.0 mg; pregnancy 1.4 mg; lactation 1.4 mg
- 19-50 years: male 1.2 mg: female 1.1 mg; pregnancy 1.4 mg; lactation 1.4 mg
- 51 plus years: male 1.2 mg: female 1.1 mg

Vitamin B2

Vitamin B2 is another water-soluble vitamin in the B complex, also known as riboflavin, which helps to breakdown proteins, fats, and carbohydrates. It also acts as an important cofactor in numerous enzyme reactions and is vital for energy production. As it is water-soluble and is carried through the bloodstream, unused quantities are excreted in the urine. We therefore need a regular and sufficient dietary intake. Food sources, include yeast extracts, eggs, dairy products, green leafy vegetables, mushrooms, and almonds. Mild deficiency is known to affect over 50% of Third World Countries, and both fortification and supplementation are used in many other countries to bridge any gaps.[93] Signs and symptoms of deficiency include: skin disorders, hyperaemia (an excess of blood in the vessels), oedema (excess fluid) in the mouth and throat, lesions at the corners of the mouth, swollen and cracked lips, hair loss, reproductive problems, a sore throat, itchy and red eyes, and degeneration of the liver and nervous system. Vitamin B2 was discovered in 1922 by German scientist, Richard Kuhn (1900-1967) and by Austrian scientist, Theodor Wagner-Jauregg (1903-1992), in the same year. The actual vitamin compound riboflavin was isolated, in Germany in 1933, by Kuhn and Paul György (1893-1976).[94] The RDA is around 1.3 mg per day for men and 1.1 mg per day for women. There are no published upper limits for riboflavin, and the full RDAs are listed below.[95]

Recommended Dietary Allowances (RDAs)

- 0-6 months: male 0.3 mg: female 0.3 mg, also AI
- 7-12 months: male 0.4 mg: female 0.4 mg, also AI
- 1-3 years: male 0.5 mg: female 0.5 mg
- 4-8 years: male 0.6 mg: female 0.6 mg
- 9-13 years: male 0.9 mg: female 0.9 mg
- 14-18 years: male 1.3 mg: female 1.0 mg; pregnancy 1.4 mg; lactation 1.6 mg
- 19-50 years: male 1.3 mg: female 1.1 mg; pregnancy 1.4 mg; lactation 1.6 mg
- 51 plus years: male 1.3 mg: female 1.1 mg

Vitamin B3

Vitamin B3, also known as niacin, niacinamide, and

nicotinamide riboside, is found in whole grains, nuts, meat and poultry, eggs, dairy products, and oily fish. All three of the compounds are required precursors for production of NAD (Nicotinamide Adenine Dinucleotide), a cofactor central to metabolic function and needing Vitamin B3 for production. NAD has a strong relationship with the essential amino acid, tryptophan, involved in immune regulation. NAD is found in every cell and is therefore vital for human metabolism. A deficiency causes the rare disease pellagra, which produces symptoms of dermatitis, diarrhoea, and dementia. It was named vitamin B3, as it was the third vitamin discovered in the B group. Again, it was the Polish-American biochemist, Casimir Funk, who in 1912 isolated nicotinic acid while he was researching beriberi, as discussed under vitamin B1. Pellagra was named as a separate disease in 1771 by an Italian doctor, Francesco Frapolli, and was especially associated with corn-based diets amongst the impoverished people of Europe. Whilst they may have eaten enough maize, we would consider the people malnourished, as corn or maize consists mainly of carbohydrate and water.[96] The RDA for vitamin B3 is around 16.5 mg per day for men and 13.2 mg per day for women. Full RDAs and ULs are listed below. NE represents niacin equivalents.[97]

Recommended Dietary Allowances (RDAs)

- 0-6 months: male 2 mg: female 2 mg, also AI (Adequate Intake)
- 7-12 months: male 4 mg NE: female 4 mg NE, also AI (Adequate Intake)
- 1-3 years: male 6 mg NE: female 6 mg NE
- 4-8 years: male 8 mg NE: female 8 mg NE
- 9-13 years: male 12 mg NE: female 12 mg NE
- 14-18 years: male 16 mg NE: female 14 mg NE; pregnancy 18 mg NE; lactation 17 mg NE
- 19 plus years: male 16 mg NE: female 14 mg NE; pregnancy 18 mg NE; lactation 17 mg NE

Tolerable upper limits vary according to age and are shown below.

Upper limits (ULs)

- 0-6 months none established
- 7-12 months none established
- 1-3 years: male 10 mg: female 10 mg
- 4-8 years: male 15 mg: female 15 mg
- 9-13 years: male 20 mg: female 20 mg
- 14-18 years: male 30 mg: female 30 mg and pregnancy and lactating both 30 mg
- 19 plus years: male 35 mg: female 35 mg and pregnancy and lactating both 35 mg

The only sources of niacin for children should come from breast milk, formula, and food.

Vitamin B5

Vitamin B5 (or pantothenic acid) is another water-soluble vitamin widely found in foods such as whole grains, eggs, nuts, yeast, and shiitake mushrooms. This vitamin is vital for numerous metabolic reactions. EFSA suggests that water-soluble vitamins, calcium, magnesium, and zinc are essential for mental function and performance. In addition, it is suggested that pantothenic acid can support a healthy hormone balance, help to fight skin dryness, and is required for normal adrenal function. The adrenal glands are located just above the kidneys and produce hormones that help regulate metabolism — they are involved with immune system function, blood pressure regulation and respond to stressors in the environment. Vitamin B5 supplementation, along with other B-vitamins, iron, magnesium, and vitamin C can reduce fatigue and tiredness in situations of inadequate micronutrient uptake.[98] Vitamin B5, was discovered in 1933 by Dr. R. J. Williams, an American biochemist, and was subsequently established as a true vitamin. The name is derived from the Greek word "pantos", meaning "everywhere"; appropriate considering its wide distribution in many foods.[99] NHS UK suggests that you need this in your diet, on a daily basis, and that taking 200 mg or less per day of pantothenic acid in supplement form is unlikely to cause any harm, but no human data has established tolerable upper limits. The full RDAs for vitamin B5 are shown below.[100]

Recommended Dietary Allowances (RDAs)

- 0-6 months: male 1.7 mg: female 1.7 mg
- 7-12 months: male 1.8 mg: female 1.8 mg
- 1-3 years: male 2 mg: female 2 mg
- 4-8 years: male 3 mg: female 3 mg
- 9-13 years: male 4 mg: female 4 mg
- 14-18 years: male 5 mg: female 5 mg; pregnancy 6 mg; lactation 7 mg
- 19 plus years: male 5 mg: female 5mg; pregnancy 6 mg; lactation 7 mg

Vitamin B6

Vitamin B6 is actually a group of water-soluble compounds, including pyridoxine, pyridoxal, and pyridoxamine. These all give rise to pyridoxine, the very active form of B6 involved with numerous vital amino acid, glucose, and lipid reactions in the body. Important food sources, include whole grains, meat, oily fish, liver, dark chocolate, potatoes, bananas, chickpeas, and pistachios. Vitamin B6 helps to maintain a normal blood level of homocysteine, a natural breakdown product of the dietary amino acid methionine. Normal levels help to maintain a healthy heart and circulation. To take place completely, this sequence of reactions also needs the presence of folic acid and vitamin B12. Symptoms and signs of deficiency include dermatitis, split lips, an inflamed tongue, neuropathy (nerve damage), symptoms of anxiety and confusion, as well as a type of anaemia. EFSA suggests it is necessary for healthy teeth, bones, hair, skin, and nails, and that vitamin B6 is also necessary for maintenance of proper energy levels and general vitality.[101] Vitamin B6 ensures normal functioning of the body`s organ tissues and systems, particularly in old age. Fortunately, deficiency is uncommon, but when present often occurs in conjunction with other vitamin B complex deficiencies. Pyridoxine was discovered in the 1930s as the result of a series of nutritional studies in rats that were fed vitamin-free diets.[102] The RDA for vitamin B6 is around 1.4 mg per day for men and 1.2 mg per day for women. The full RDAs and ULs for vitamin B6 are shown below.[103]

Recommended Dietary Allowances (RDAs)

- 0-6 months: male 0.1 mg: female 0.1 mg, AI (adequate intake)
- 7-12 months: male 0.3 mg: female 0.3 mg, AI
- 1-3 years: male 0.5 mg: female 0.5 mg
- 4-8 years: male 0.6 mg: female 0.6 mg
- 9-13 years: male 1.0 mg: female 1.0 mg
- 14-18 years: male 1.3 mg: female 1.2 mg; pregnancy 1.9 mg; lactation 2.0 mg
- 19-50 years: male 1.3 mg: female 1.3 mg; pregnancy 1.9 mg; lactation 2.0 mg
- 51 years plus: male 1.7 mg: female 1.5 mg

Tolerable upper limits vary according to age and are shown below for vitamin B6.

Upper limits (ULs)

- 0-6 months: none has been possible to establish
- 7-12 months: none has been possible to establish
- 1-3 years: male 30 mg: female 30 mg

- 4-8 years: male 40 mg: female 40 mg
- 9-13 years: male 60 mg: female 60 mg
- 14-18 years: male 80 mg: female 80 mg and pregnancy and lactating both 80 mg
- 19 plus years: male 100 mg: female 100 mg and pregnancy and lactating both 100 mg

Vitamin B12

Vitamin B12 (also known as cobalamin) is a water-soluble compound containing cobalt, a fundamental cofactor in the synthesis of DNA (Deoxyribonucleic acid) — the hereditary code of life. We can obtain vitamin B12 from a wide range of animal products, fish, and eggs. Absorption of this essential vitamin is facilitated by an intrinsic factor, a glycoprotein found in the stomach. A failure in production or utilisation of this protein can lead to deficiency. As we get older, a decline in gastric acid production can also contribute to deficiency through malabsorption. This has the potential to lead to the disease pernicious anaemia, a disease characterised by an increase in the numbers of some circulating large blood cell types, leading to various neurological symptoms, both peripheral and central in nature. EFSA considers a wide range of health benefits related to proper vitamin B12 absorption, such as normal mental function and cognition, particularly as we get older.[104] Vitamin B12 was one of the last real vitamins to be classified. It was finally isolated from liver extracts in 1948 by two chemists, Karl Folkers and Alexander Todd. The actual chemical structure was later elucidated by Dorothy Hodgkin, a British chemist, in 1956. As a result, this allowed for new methods of synthesis from the late 1950s onwards.[105] It is suggested that adults need about 1.5 micrograms (mcg) of vitamin B12 per day. The full RDAs are shown below.[106]

Recommended Dietary Allowances (RDAs)

- 0-6 months: male 0.4 mcg: female 0.4 mcg, AI
- 7-12 months: male 0.5 mcg: female 0.5 mcg, AI
- 1-3 years: male 0.9 mcg: female 0.9 mcg
- 4-8 years: male 1.2 mcg: female 1.2 mcg
- 9-13 years: male 1.8 mcg: female 1.8 mcg
- 14 plus years: male 2.4 mcg: female 2.4 mcg; pregnancy 2.6 mcg; lactation 2.8 mcg

No tolerable upper intake levels have been established for vitamin B12, as little research exists to corroborate high levels and any association with harm.[107]

Baobab- Adansonia digitata

The baobab tree is found in the arid regions of Africa, Arabia, and Australia. It is a prehistoric species, predating both mankind and the splitting of the continents over 200 million years ago. Some believe the trees can live for nearly 5,000 years, reaching 30 metres in height, with gigantic circumferences of up to 50 metres. The trees provide shelter, food, and water to animals and humans alike.[108] There are nine species of this tree, six of which are found in Madagascar, and one individual African tree was aged at 1,275 years old by carbon-14 dating. Recently some older specimens have been dying prematurely and this may be attributable to climate change.[109] Both the fruits and leaves are edible and have been used in herbal remedies for centuries. The fruits themselves are a good source of vitamin C, potassium, and phosphorus, and like many fruits are good sources of carbohydrates.

Barberry- Berberis vulgaris

The common barberry is a shrub that can grow to sixteen feet tall, with a wide variety of species found in temperate and subtropical regions across the entire world. Extracts, particularly from the roots, rhizomes, and stem bark contain the compound berberine, which has been shown to increase insulin sensitivity (insulin is an important hormone produced in the pancreas, which is important for regulating blood sugar levels) and can improve the function of some liver enzymes involved with modulating cholesterol density in blood serum.[110] However, some studies have shown that berberine interacts adversely with some prescription drugs, and that at certain levels might even be toxic.[111]

Beetroot- Beta vulgaris

The raw root of beetroot is rich in folate, also known as vitamin B9, and is a moderate source of manganese. The leaves are also eaten and are known as beet leaves. Taken as a supplement with inorganic nitrate, it was found to be associated with the lowering of blood pressure.[112] Sugar beet comes from the same family as beetroot (Amaranthaceae), but is a genetically different plant. The sugar beet is white in colour and has a higher sucrose content, so is frequently used in sugar production.

Berberine

Berberine is an ammonium salt found in a variety of plants, which include the European barberry (see above), goldenseal, Oregon grape, tree turmeric, goldenseal, yellow root, and Chinese goldthread. Research has shown that it could be effective for treating canker sores when applied topically and has shown significant antimicrobial properties against many microorganisms. Berberine also seems to slightly lower blood sugar levels in people with diabetes and might help to lower cholesterol in people with high blood levels.[113]

Bifidobacterium

These are a group of bacteria that live in the human intestines and stomach, and include varieties such as breve, longum, infantis, and bifidus. These bacteria are part of our microbiota and play an important role in carbohydrate fermentation. Improved rates of remission and maintenance, in ulcerative colitis sufferers, have been shown when the bacteria are ingested, and used in conjunction with conventional treatments,[114] but most evidence suggests that Bifidobacterium, by itself, is not beneficial for preventing any relapses. They are considered key commensals (organisms, such as many bacteria that can provide the host — humans and other animals — with essential nutrients), working symbiotically to promote a healthy gastrointestinal tract.[115] There are several additional possible benefits. Airway infections, such as the common cold, are reduced in otherwise healthy people, including school children and college students. There may be a shortening of the duration of diarrhoea in infants with rotavirus (a highly infectious stomach bug), and a reduction in irritable bowel syndrome (IBS) symptoms, including stomach pains, bloating, and constipation. Bifidobacterium may also reduce symptoms of anxiety and depression in sufferers of IBS.[116]

Bilberry- Vaccinium myrtillus

This bush is related to the blueberry, blackcurrant, and grape, and is native to many regions, including the Rocky Mountains, and large areas of Europe and Asia. It is referred to colloquially as a whortleberry or huckleberry, and its dark blue berries and leaves have been used extensively since the Middle Ages for treating a variety of conditions. These include scurvy, infections, burns, and diabetes. During World War II, British pilots ate bilberry jam in the hope that it would improve their night vision, possibly because its berries contained high levels of antioxidants called anthocyanins. There is evidence that the anthocyanins found in the berries, especially the compounds called delphinidins and cyanidins, are both bioavailable (can enter the circulation when introduced into the body) and bioactive (able to have an active physiological effect), leading to a variety of health benefits.[117] No strong scientific evidence is available to support the use of bilberry for any specific health conditions, but the bilberry is still of great interest to researchers, with some ongoing studies investigating the effects of its antioxidant content.[118]

Biotin

Biotin is a water-soluble vitamin, also called vitamin H, vitamin B7 or vitamin B8. It is important for the metabolism of fatty acids, amino acids, and carbohydrates. Biotin is also required to maintain healthy teeth, bones, hair, skin, and nails.[119] Deficiency can occur by consuming raw egg whites daily for several months, as the proteins bind to the vitamin, thus making absorption difficult. Cooked egg white does not have the same effect. Symptoms of deficiency can include — brittle nails, reversible hair loss, conjunctivitis, and skin irritation, tiredness, numbness and tingling in the extremities, depression, muscle pain, and wasting. Adequate intakes vary with age. Higher quantities are required during pregnancy and lactation, with 35 mcg representing the daily recommended requirement during these stages.[120] NHS UK suggests that taking 0.9 mg or lower quantities per day, in supplements, is unlikely to cause any harm.[121] The Adequate Intakes (AIs) are shown below, as insufficient data was found to support Estimated Average Requirements (EARs) or Recommended Dietary Allowances (RDAs) for biotin.[122]

Adequate Intakes (AIs)

- 0-6 months: male 5 mcg: female 5 mcg
- 7-12 months: male 6 mcg: female 6 mcg

- 1-3 years: male 8 mcg: female 8 mcg
- 4-8 years: male 12 mcg: female 12 mcg
- 9-13 years: male 20 mcg: female 20 mcg
- 14-18 years: male 25 mcg: female 25 mcg; pregnancy 30 mcg; lactation 35 mcg
- 19 plus years: male 30 mcg: female 30 mcg; pregnancy 30 mcg; lactation 35 mcg

Bitter Orange- Citrus aurantium

This is a citrus tree with a bitter tasting fruit, thought to be a cross between a pomelo and Mandarin orange, sometimes known as a Seville or bigarade orange. The tree is grown throughout the Mediterranean region, also in California and Florida. However, it was originally native to eastern Africa, the Arabian Peninsula, and Southeast Asia. Traditionally it was used in Chinese medicine to treat indigestion, nausea, and constipation. The active ingredient is called p-synephrine, which is similar to the main chemical in the herb, ephedra, but has different properties. Ephedra, itself, is banned from dietary substances in the US. Topical application of bitter orange oil extracts may help with ringworm, jock itch, and athlete`s foot, but there is insufficient evidence to demonstrate efficacy for weight loss or any other health claims.[123]

Blackcurrants- Ribes nigrum

Blackcurrant is a woody shrub with berries that are rich in vitamin C, iron, and manganese. It has been used for centuries in traditional herbal medicine, with many anecdotal health benefits. More recent in-vitro studies have shown the potent anti-inflammatory, antioxidant, and antimicrobial effects of some blackberry constituents on many disease states.[124] Blackcurrant seeds also contain vitamin E and fatty acids. The oil extracts appear promising for helping some critically ill patients who are unable to convert linoleic acid, an essential omega-6 fatty acid, into other fatty acid compounds.[125]

Black Cohosh- Actaea racemosa & Cimicifuga racemosa

This plant is a member of the buttercup family, native to North America; its root or rhizome has traditionally been used to treat a variety of ailments, by both Native Americans and Chinese herbalists. It has also been used as an insect repellent, as it has a foetid odour that repels bugs, but still attracts butterflies; it was named bugwort and bugbane as a result. A 2016 systematic review concluded there were no significant associations between supplementation with black cohosh and any reduction in the number of vasomotor symptoms, such as hot flushes or other menopausal symptoms, in women. Nevertheless, a Cochrane review found adequate justification for conducting further studies into the treatment or alleviation of menopausal symptoms. Its authors also recommended conducting higher quality trials with larger sample sizes.[126]

Black Garlic

Black garlic is obtained from fresh garlic -Allium sativum-, and through fermentation loses the pungency of fresh garlic. Consequently, it is mildly scented and has a different taste, sometimes compared to a slightly sour or bitter caramel, but still retains an enhanced bioactivity when compared to fresh garlic. Black garlic is being investigated for its potential health benefits, which may include protective effects against the pathogenesis of diabetes mellitus.[127] The active component under investigation is a garlic derivative, S-allylcysteine (SAC). SAC also exhibits a considerable number of positive actions in cell models and living systems, and in addition, the compound may have certain neuroprotective and anti-inflammatory properties.[128]

Black Pepper- Piper nigrum

Black pepper plants are cultivated for the peppercorn fruits, which grow in clumps on a flowering vine. They have been widely used in cooking since ancient times, when it was known as black gold as it was so highly prized. It is thought to be the world's most commonly used spice, originally native to southern India, with archaeological evidence of people using pepper over 4,000 years ago.[129] More recently, we have found that by removing the outer skin, peppercorns have a more delicate flavour, as well as a higher bioactivity due to the retention of the active compound piperine. This is the alkaloid responsible for the pungent flavour of black pepper. Piperine has also been found to increase the bioavailability of other useful compounds such as curcumin. Curcumin is found in turmeric, a flowering plant and an ancient Indian herb related to ginger, which may have some promising health benefits itself.[130] We often see compounds working together in this synergistic fashion. These interactions are worth exploring further.

Black tea

This is a beverage made from the Camellia sinensis plant, a flowering shrub or small tree. This plant species and the assamica variety are used in other aromatic teas, including white, yellow, green, oolong, and dark teas. Black tea uses aged leaves and stems, and might be effective for improving mental alertness, for lowering blood pressure and associated risks of heart disease. It might also be associated with lower risks of hip fractures in the elderly, lowered risks of developing ovarian cancer in women who regularly drink tea, and some research shows that the caffeine found in a wide variety of beverages, including coffee, cola, and tea might even lower the risk of Parkinson`s disease under certain circumstances.[131] Parkinson`s disease is a progressive nervous system disorder that affects movement and causes problems such as shaking and stiffness. The other active ingredients in black tea that are probably responsible for the claimed effects, apart from increasing mental alertness, are the polyphenols, particularly the flavonoids.

Blueberry- Vaccinium corymbosum

The blueberry is a North American species of perennial flowering plant with purple or blue coloured berries. It is rich in the essential mineral manganese, vitamin C, vitamin K, and has small amounts of other vitamins, with some dietary fibre content too. Blueberries also contain anthocyanins, other polyphenols, and a variety of phytochemicals. Some of these are under ongoing preliminary research for the roles they may play in the human body. A 2019 paper looking at a variety of epidemiological studies (epidemiology is the branch of medicine which deals with the incidence, distribution, and possible control of diseases, and other factors relating to health)[132] associated regular moderate intake of blueberries with a reduced risk of cardiovascular disease and type 2 diabetes, as well as improved weight maintenance and neuroprotection. These findings are supported by biomarker-based evidence from human studies. Blueberries exhibit anti-inflammatory and antioxidant properties due to their polyphenol content, and the phytochemicals may also help the constitution of the human microbiome, thereby contributing to our systemic health.[133]

Borage- Borago officinalis

Borage is also known as the star flower and was originally native to the Mediterranean, but now grows quite widely as a self-seeding plant. Along with other members of the Boraginaceae family of plants, such as comfrey, it is one of the favourite foods of scarlet tiger moth caterpillars. Many European people are also fond of eating both the leaves and flowers. In Italy it is a popular ingredient used for the fillings in ravioli and pansoti.[134] Borage has been used traditionally to treat hyperactive gastrointestinal, respiratory, and cardiovascular disorders, and extracts have also shown promise as antispasmodics.[135] The seeds are used to produce oils, which are the richest known source of gamma-linolenic acid (GLA), also containing a number of other fatty acids, including the essential linoleic acid (LA). We have lost the ability to synthesise LA, but GLA itself can be made from LA (please see the omega-6 fatty acid entry).[136] Care needs to be taken during the processing of Borage oil as extracts contain small amounts of liver toxic compounds, known as Pyrrolizidine alkaloids.[137]

Broccoli- Brassica oleracea

Broccoli is a dark green edible plant with a slightly bitter flavour, which is another brassica, part of the cabbage family. Broccoli may have been known to the Greeks up to 2,500 years ago, but the modern varieties arose in Italy during the last 2,000 years or so.[138] Broccoli is a mid-17th century word derived from Italian, the plural of "broccolo", meaning "cabbage sprout/head".[139] An English derivation of the word may go back many centuries to a Proto-Celtic word "brokkos", meaning badger; the reason is unknown.[140] Broccoli is a rich source of vitamins C and K, and also contains folate, manganese, and other minerals, and surprisingly carotenoids that tend to give other plants a yellow-orange colour.

Butterbur- Petasides hybridus and officinalis *also* Tussilago hybrid

Butterbur is a shrub that likes wet marshy ground and grows in Europe, parts of Asia, and North America. The name is thought to relate to a traditional use of its large leaves, which were used to wrap butter when the weather was warm, presumably because the leaves were large and pliable; these were the days before refrigeration. The active ingredients in this marsh-loving shrub, pentasin and isopetasin, have been linked to a reduction in the frequency of migraine attacks in sufferers, and extracts have also shown promise for relieving the symptoms of hay fever. It has been used since the Middle Ages for plague and fever symptoms, and into the 17th century, it was used to treat coughs, asthma, and skin wounds.[141] In 2018, based upon two high-quality studies, The American Headache Society endorsed butterbur extracts, made from the underground parts of the plant, for migraine prevention in some sufferers. Several other over-the-counter preparations containing feverfew, magnesium, vitamin B2, coenzyme Q10, and melatonin have been shown, in randomised controlled trials, to help with migraines, and these were validated by the same society too.[142] Regarding safety, the raw unprocessed butterbur plant contains chemicals called pyrrolizidine alkaloids (PAs), also found in borage, which can cause liver damage, consequently resulting in serious illness. So, only butterbur products, which are appropriately labelled, and have been processed to remove PAs, should be consumed — but not during pregnancy or by breastfeeding women. In April 2019, an article concluded that butterbur was generally well tolerated and its efficacy in treating seasonal allergic rhinitis symptoms was comparable to several over-the-counter antihistamines. However, patients with allergies to ragweed should also avoid usage.[143] Ragweed (Ambrosia) pollen is the main culprit in up to 50% of all cases of pollinosis (hay fever in response to pollen generally) in North America. There have been increasing concerns in Switzerland, where up to 12% of the population suffer from allergies to ragweed, which was beginning to invade the country back in the year 2005, and this will require diligant, ongoing surveillance.[144]

C

Vitamin C

Vitamin C is a water-soluble vitamin that cannot be stored in the body in large quantities. It is also known as ascorbic acid, fulfilling many vital functions in the human body, including — helping to protect cells from damage and assisting with wound healing, as well as maintaining healthy skin, bones, cartilage, and blood vessels. We need sufficient vitamin C in our diets to avoid scurvy, a disease with a range of symptoms, including lethargy, bone pain, bleeding gums, and poor wound healing. Left untreated scurvy will lead to convulsions and eventually death. Research has also shown that whilst vitamin C does not cure the common cold it can reduce its duration.[145] Vitamin C is found in a wide range of fruits and vegetables, including broccoli, potatoes, blackcurrants, kale, sea buckthorn, citrus fruits, and capsicums — to name just a few. Many animals can make their own vitamin C. Unfortunately, humans cannot, and nor can other anthropoid primates, guinea pigs or bats, teleost fishes, and Passeriformes bird species — perching birds. All these species have lost the capacity to synthesise vitamin C; a strange quirk of evolution.[146] Adults require around 40 mg per day. Whilst we should be able to get all we need from our diets, taking less than 1,000 mg of vitamin C supplements per day should cause no harm, according to NHS UK.[147] Vitamin C is an antioxidant that protects cells in the body, by acting against age-accelerating free radicals. Vitamin C also contributes to iron absorption from food, helps the nervous system to work correctly, and is needed for normal mental function. Vitamin C helps to support the immune system, which is depressed during exercise, and is therefore an important compound for the body`s defences. Vitamin C is also vitally important for energy metabolism, collagen formation, protection of the eyes from oxidative stress, and the health of the retina and lens that become damaged over the years by sunlight, smoke, and pollution. Vitamin C promotes lutein and zeaxanthin, two carotenoids that filter out harmful blue wavelengths of light, which can damage cells in the eyes. [148] The National Institute of Health (US) RDAs are shown below,[149] and are generally higher than the UK RDAs, although these are still under review. The amounts that prevent scurvy may not be sufficient to optimally protect against, or reduce the risk of, chronic diseases such as cancer, cardiovascular, and cataracts. The totality of reviewed data indicates a possible new RDA of around 120 mg per day.[150]

Recommended Dietary Allowances (RDAs)

- 0-6 months: male 40 mg: female 40 mg, also AI (Adequate Intake)
- 7-12 months: male 50 mg: female 50 mg, also AI
- 1-3 years: male 15 mg: female 15 mg
- 4-8 years: male 25 mg: female 25 mg
- 9-13 years: male 45 mg: female 45 mg
- 14-18 years: male 75 mg: female 65 mg; pregnancy 80 mg; lactation 115 mg
- 19 plus years: male 90 mg: female 75 mg; pregnancy 85 mg; lactation 120 mg

Tolerable upper limits vary according to age and are shown below for vitamin C.

Upper limits (ULs)

- 0-12 months: none has been possible to establish
- 1-3 years: male 400 mg: female 400 mg
- 4-8 years: male 650 mg: female 650 mg
- 9-13 years: male 1,200 mg: female 1,200 mg
- 14-18 years: male 1,800 mg: female 1,800 mg; and pregnancy and lactating both 1,800 mg
- 19 plus years: male 2,000 mg: female 2,000 mg; and pregnancy and lactating both 2,000 mg

Calcium-Ca

This is one of the essential elements with atomic number 20. Calcium is vital for building strong bones and teeth, making sure that blood clots normally, and regulating muscle contractions, including cardiac muscle. Insufficient calcium in the diet can lead to rickets in children, and later in life — osteomalacia (a softening of bones), or osteoporosis (where the bones become brittle and fragile) — associated with an increased risk of fractures. If you are at all concerned about your own fracture risk, there is an online Fracture Risk Assessment Tool (FRAX).[151] Dietary sources of calcium, include dairy products, soya beans, nuts, and fish, such as sardines, salmon, and pilchards, also green leafy vegetables. Spinach is an exception, as it contains oxalate compounds, which hinder calcium absorption from the gut. Adults require around 700 mg per day. Full US-based RDAs and ULs for calcium are shown below.[152]

Recommended Dietary Allowances (RDAs)

- 0-6 months: male 200 mg: female 200 mg, also AI (Adequate Intake)
- 7-12 months: male 260 mg: female 260 mg, also AI
- 1-3 years: male 700 mg: female 700 mg
- 4-8 years: male 1,000 mg: female 1,000 mg
- 9-13 years: male 1,300 mg: female 1,300 mg
- 14-18 years: male 1,300 mg: female 1,300 mg; pregnancy

- 1,300 mg; lactation 1,300 mg
- 19-50 years: male 1,000 mg: female 1,000 mg; pregnancy 1,000 mg; lactation 1,000 mg
- 51-70 years: male 1,000 mg: female 1,200 mg
- 71 plus years: male 1,200 mg: female 1,200 mg

Tolerable upper limits or upper intake levels vary according to age and are shown below for calcium, which are also associated with vitamin D levels.[153]

Upper limits (ULs)

- 0-6 months: male 1,000 mg: female 1,000 mg
- 7-12 months: male 1,500 mg: female 1,500 mg
- 1-8 years: male 2,500 mg: female 2,500 mg
- 9-18 years: male 3,000 mg: female 3,000 mg; pregnant and lactating both 3,000 mg
- 19-50 years: male 2,500 mg: female 2,500 mg; pregnant and lactating both 2,500 mg
- 51 years plus: male 2,000 mg: female 2,000 mg

Cannabidiol

Cannabidiol (CBD) is an extract derived from the Cannabis sativa plant. Records show that the plant itself has been used variously, as a source of industrial fibre, oil, as a food, and for recreation; it is often used in religious ceremonies and within spiritual settings. Cannabis or marijuana contains over 80 compounds, but delta-9-tetrahydrocannabinol (THC) is the major active ingredient, the main psychoactive compound found in marijuana that is prohibited for recreational use in most countries — Malta, however, recently became the first country in the European Union to assent to the use and growing of marijuana for recreational purposes. Hemp extracts containing less than 0.3 % THC, together with the compound CBD, are used in various proprietary gels, oils, supplements, and extracts. CBD is considered effective in the treatment of epilepsy, particularly in a paediatric setting,[154] but is not approved for treating all types of seizures.

Capsaicin

Capsaicin is an active compound found in chilli peppers, members of the Capsicum genus; the chemical, capsaicin, derived from the fruits and seeds, is responsible for the burning sensation experienced upon contact. It is a discomforting irritant for mammals, including humans. It is also, conversely in a way, the component of chilli peppers, which many people enjoy worldwide. The pungency of chillis is measured on the Scoville scale, named after an American pharmacist, Wilbur Scoville, in 1912. A Bell pepper might have a value up to around 100 units on this scale, Cayenne pepper around 50,000 units, and the Naga viper pepper, one on the hottest chillis in the world, registers around 1,359,000 units on the scale. This is considered hot enough to strip paint.[155] The 2013 Guinness World Records named the Carolina Reaper the hottest chilli in the world, with one example reaching a staggering 2,200,000 Scoville Heat Units.[156] This positions the Reaper just below most, not all, US law enforcement pepper spray values, which are often used by police forces to control or disperse crowds. Research shows that chilli pepper plants may have developed their heat to fight off fungal infections caused by insects. This is another example of a phytochemical protecting a plant from pathogen invasion.[157] According to some studies and considered acceptable health claims by EFSA, capsaicin enhances the loss of calories, burns carbohydrates, burns fats, helps to maintain a healthy lipid profile, reduces calorific intake, and helps to promote hair growth.[158] Capsicums (chilli peppers) are considered beneficial in treating nerve pain linked to diabetic neuropathy, when used as a cream or patch, and can also give temporary relief from the chronic pain associated with shingles (this pain is known as postherpetic neuralgia).[159]

Carotenoids

We have often discussed this group of organic pigments, which have a yellow or orange hue, on account of their health benefits and prevalence in the plant kingdom. A number of studies have investigated these possible benefits, with one 2015 review finding that carotenoids appeared to be involved in a reduction of the rates of mouth and neck cancer.[160] Another review showed a possible link with prostate cancer inhibition.[161] Several studies have shown positive improvements in skin quality.[162] Carotenoids are generally found in richly pigmented plants and fruits, such as carrots, tomatoes, sweet potatoes, broccoli, and kale. Some carotenoids, including beta-carotene, can be converted into the essential vitamin A or retinol, which both protects the eyes and supports a healthy immune system.

Caraway- Carum carvi

Caraway, also known as Persian cumin, is a member of the carrot family. The fruits have a pungent anise flavour and aroma derived from its essential oils — limonene and carvone. These aromatic oils are also found in spearmint, dill, citrus fruit peels, anise, fennel, and liquorice. The seeds contain vitamins B1, B2, B3, B6, C, and E, and the minerals calcium, magnesium, phosphorus, potassium, zinc, with high levels of iron. Caraway has and is still used as a spice in rye bread, some desserts, liquors, casseroles (such as goulash), and as a cheese flavouring. Finland is one of the World`s largest exporters, with between 20 and 30 percent, by volume, of the global production share. Finland has a very long growing season, with light-filled days, and this increases the quantity and quality of essential oils in the seeds when compared to caraway seeds sourced from other countries. This in turn generates a much stronger flavour.[163]

Cascara sagrada- Rhamnus purshiana

This shrub is native to North America and parts of Canada, often used by indigenous peoples for its laxative properties. Today the bark is dried and then used, and research shows it may be effective for relieving constipation. The fruits are sometimes referred to as bear berries. The active chemicals thought responsible for the laxative effects are called hydroxyanthracene glycosides and emodins, and they are thought to work by increasing gut motility.[164] Emodins are compounds that can also be isolated from rhubarb, buckthorn, and Japanese knotweed. These compounds have been shown to have anticancer properties in several in-vitro and animal studies.[165]

Cat`s Claw- Uncaria tomentosa, Uncaria guianensis

Cat`s claw is a woody vine that grows wild in the tropical rainforests of the Amazon and other equatorial areas of Central and South America. Its name is derived from its thorns, which resemble cat`s claws. The Spanish translation for cat`s claw is "Una de gato", which is the common name for at least another 20 species of plants. The two described here are the most common varieties used in commercial preparations, namely U.tomentosa and U.guianensis, each having different properties and uses.[166] The Inca civilisation is known to have used cat`s claw for contraception, as an anti-inflammatory, to treat cancer, and viral infections, also to stimulate or invigorate the immune system. The bark and roots have been used to make extracts, capsules, tablets, and teas, but very few high-quality studies have been conducted that support any health uses. Cat`s claw is deemed to be safe, with very few reported side effects, but best avoided in women who are pregnant or trying to become pregnant.[167]

Cauliflower- Brassica oleracea

Cauliflower is an annual plant belonging to the brassica genus, which contains high levels of vitamin C and several protective phytochemicals. It is considered a moderate source of vitamins B5, B6, B9, and K, also housing a wide spectrum of minerals. The cauliflower is a close relative of broccoli, originally hailing from Cyprus. The Roman writer Pliny the Elder valued its pleasant taste back in the first century AD, when it was known as "cyma", but the modern cultivated forms were, quite likely, developed in the late Middle Ages and early Renaissance periods. It seems to have been unknown in England until around 1720, when it was called "sprout cauliflower" or "Italian asparagus".[168]

Chamomile- Anthemis nobilis Matricaria recutita, Chamomilla recutita

There are two species of these daisy-like flowering herbs, which are used today in supplements for anxiety, gastrointestinal conditions, skin conditions, and mouth sores resulting from certain cancer treatments. They are colloquially called German chamomile and Roman chamomile. Extracts from the flowering tops of German chamomile (Chamomilla recutita) have been investigated in some preliminary studies, which have suggested that chamomile may be helpful for treating generalised anxiety disorder (GAD). Some other research has found a combination of herbs, also containing chamomile, might be beneficial for gastrointestinal upset, diarrhoea in children, and for infants suffering with colic.[169] This popular relation of the daisy contains antioxidant polyphenols and terpenoids that have demonstrable health benefits in some animal studies, but there is a paucity of research in humans.[170] A 2020 systematic review into the effects of chamomile in diabetes mellitus concluded that both sugar status and oxidative stress might be improved in patients, but acknowledged that findings were contradictory from different papers.[171]

Chicory- Cichorium intybus

Chicory is a member of the dandelion family, also known as an endive. It is grown in complete darkness, as a forced crop, to make it slightly sweeter, and this accounts for its white or light-yellow-tipped leaves. The crisp leaves are usually considered mildly bitter or sharp in flavour. Chicory root contains inulin, a sweetener used in the food industry, and the leaves themselves have good nutritional value. They contain vitamins A, B, with a high vitamin K content — 100 g of chicory representing 215% of our Daily Value.[172] The leaves also contain minerals, including potassium, calcium, copper, and manganese. It has been used since ancient Egyptian times as a food and medicine, and more recently roasted and added to coffee. It became extremely popular in 19th century France because of its similar flavour to coffee — it is also caffeine free.[173]

Chinese herbal medicine

There are many similarities between traditional Chinese Herbal Medicine (CHM) and Ayurvedic Indian medicine. Both philosophies embrace exercise and lifestyle, as well as using herbs for both medicinal and food purposes. Regarding exercise, the Chinese form of meditatory movements is known as tai chi; this was originally created as a fighting art many centuries ago. Even older, some think up to 5,000 years, is an Indian version of meditatory exercise known as yoga. This also involves slow considered movements and stretching; it is not a martial art though! Additionally, the Chinese adopted a traditional medicinal practice using needles, called acupuncture, to treat a wide range of ailments. Many Chinese herbal products and concoctions have been studied for efficacy. The quality of ingredients used is vital, but unfortunately some products have been found to contain contaminants. Nevertheless, one Chinese herbal plant (Artemisia annua, also known as sweet wormwood) was found to contain chemical compounds, the precursors of which were incorporated in the drug Artemisinin. It was discovered in 1972, and this drug has been widely used to treat malaria (a protozoan parasite found in humans). According to the World Health Organization (WHO), malaria killed 405,000 people in 2018, with a mighty estimate of 228 million cases of malaria experienced worldwide in the same year.[174] Other herbal combinations may also have efficacy, but the research paradigms used to assess CHM, as a facet of traditional Chinese medicine, are not well designed for the purpose. One article investigating CHM suggested that contemporary narratives should be shifted from physician-based to patient-based perspectives, to both preserve the medical tradition and its ethnic identity.[175] Herbs commonly used in CHM include: astragalus, ginkgo biloba, cinnamon, ginger, ginseng, gotu kola, rice yeasts, and yu xing cao. As discussed in the Ayurveda entry, ginger has been widely used in traditional Indian medicine, and one 2013 study using a mixture of four Indian herbs, including ginger root (Zingiber officinale), significantly reduced knee pain and improved knee function in sufferers of osteoarthritis. Chinese ginger (Boesenbergia rotunda), also known as fingerroot and lesser galangal, belongs to the same family as Zingiber officinale, namely Zingiberaceae, which contains nearly 50 genera, and approximately 1,600 known species. This aromatic tuberous rhizome is found widely across Asia, Africa, and the Americas. Not all Chinese herbs have been studied independently, or even in conjunction with other herbs, in very many well-constructed Randomised Controlled Trials (RCTs). However, under the ginger entry there is an overview of systematic reviews citing some of the other medicinal benefits of ginger itself, which contains various phenolic oily resin-like compounds, such as gingerol and gingerdiol. These last two compounds are the primary pungent ingredients believed to be responsible for a variety of remarkable pharmacological and physiological effects; currently the mechanisms of action are not fully understood.[176] This 2019 overview of systematic reviews concluded that ginger was thought to be beneficial for pain, nausea, and vomiting. It is also considered helpful for metabolic syndrome — a term for the combination of diabetes, high blood pressure, and obesity.

Chlorine-Cl

This element has atomic number 17 and is often used to reduce numbers of bacteria and viruses in water. Chloride, the negative anion of chlorine, is a component of numerous vital compounds used in the human body. Most chloride is derived from our diets in the form of salt, sodium chloride, and is important for regulating cell fluid balance, maintaining blood volume, blood pressure, and the pH of body fluids.[177] Chloride is part of the acid in our stomach known as hydrochloric acid, which is required for the breakdown of proteins, as well as providing some antimicrobial protection.[178]

Choline

Choline is an essential nutrient that must be obtained from dietary sources. It was first discovered in 1862 by Adolph Strecker, a German chemist, but its importance was not fully elucidated until the mid-1990s through controlled studies in humans.[179] As an essential nutrient, there is another aspect to the choline narrative; the bacteria in our gut microbiome like to feast on choline, which means we can easily become deficient unless we consume enough in our diets on a regular basis. Choline is a multifaceted compound. It helps to transport fat away from the liver and supports nerve impulse transmission. It also helps with brain function, particularly with cognition and memory. Choline is essential for normal brain and nervous system development, also supporting a healthy heart.[180] EFSA (The European Food Safety Authority) recommended daily requirement varies from about 140 to 520 mg per day, depending on age, with higher amounts required during pregnancy and when breastfeeding. Foods that contain high amounts of choline, include cooked bacon, beef and chicken livers, cooked pork loin, canned shrimp, broccoli, Brussels sprouts, cauliflower, peas, raw oat bran, toasted wheat germ, eggs, soybean, and avocado. The adequate intakes (AIs) and upper limits (ULs) for choline are shown below.[181]

Adequate Intakes (AIs)

- 0-6 months: male 125 mg: female 125 mg
- 7-12 months: male 150 mg: female 150 mg
- 1-3 years: male 200 mg: female 200 mg
- 4-8 years: male 250 mg: female 250 mg
- 9-13 years: male 375 mg: female 375 mg
- 14-18 years: male 550 mg: female 400 mg; pregnancy 450 mg; lactation 550 mg
- 19 plus years: male 550 mg: female 425 mg; pregnancy 450 mg; lactation 550 mg

The tolerable upper limits or upper intake levels for choline vary according to age and are shown below.

Upper limits (ULs)

- 0-12 months: not possible to establish
- 1-3 years: male 1,000 mg: female 1,000 mg
- 4-8 years: male 1,000 mg: female 1,000 mg
- 9-13 years: male 2,000 mg: female 2,000 mg
- 14-18 years: male 3,000 mg: female 3,000 mg; pregnant and lactating both 3,000 mg
- 19 years plus: male 3,500 mg: female 3,500 mg; pregnant and lactating both 3,500 mg

The only sources of choline for children 0-12 months should come from breast milk, formula, and food.

Chromium-Cr

Chromium is an element with atomic number 24. The European Food Safety Authority (EFSA) do not believe chromium is essential. Australia, New Zealand, India, Japan, and the US do though! What we do know is that chromium influences how insulin works in the body, which might affect "energy processing" of food. Chromium is found in meat, wholegrains, lentils, broccoli, potatoes, cinnamon, ginger, and cumin. We generally consume enough in our diets to achieve the daily requirement of around 25 micrograms (mcg). Adequate intakes (AIs) for chromium are shown below, as accurate RDAs could not be calculated.[182]

Daily requirements or Adequate Intakes (AIs)

- 0-6 months: male 0.2 mcg: female 0.2 mcg
- 7-12 months: male 5.5 mcg: female 5.5 mcg
- 1-3 years: male 11 mcg: female 11 mcg
- 4-8 years: male 15 mcg: female 15 mcg
- 9-13 years: male 25 mcg: female 21 mcg
- 14-18 years: male 35 mcg: female 24 mcg; pregnancy 29 mcg; lactation 44 mcg
- 19-50 years: male 35 mcg: female 25 mcg; pregnancy 30 mcg; lactation 45 mcg
- > than 50 years: male 30 mcg: female 20 mcg

High intakes of chromium have not been shown to be harmful, so no "Tolerable Upper Intake Levels" have been set for this particular mineral.

Cinquefoil- Potentilla reptans

Cinquefoil is a perennial flowering plant belonging to the rose family. The common name derives from Old French and means "five leaved", although some have 3 or 7 leaves. Most of the species, nearly three hundred, are native to the north temperate zones and Arctic regions of the planet.[183] Cinquefoil has been used in traditional herbal medicine to treat inflammation and ulcers. Tormentil, a close relative, has been studied for its possible use in treating ulcerative colitis too.[184]

Cinnamon- Cinnamomum verum

Cinnamon is an aromatic spice sourced from the inner bark of various tree species native to China, Indonesia, and Vietnam. The true or original cinnamon is from Sri Lanka and is known as Ceylon or Ceylonese cinnamon. It has been used in cuisines across the world for centuries and was thought to possess medicinal properties, most often used by sufferers of bronchitis. Several animal studies have shown that cinnamon may be effective for blood sugar control. However, very few high-quality studies in humans support cinnamon use for any health conditions, particularly with reference to glycaemic (blood sugar) control in either type 1 or type 2 diabetes — according to a Cochrane systematic review conducted in 2012.[185]

Cloves- Syzygium aromaticum

Cloves are the fragrant flower buds of a tree native to the Maluku Islands in Indonesia, commonly used as a spice in global cuisine. They are harvested in Indonesia, India, Pakistan, Sri Lanka, as well as various African countries, then exported around the world. Medicinally, they are thought to help in the control of nausea and vomiting, coughs, and diarrhoea, and have some anti-inflammatory properties too. Additionally, cloves can relieve some gastrointestinal symptoms, such as pain associated with spasms, bloating, and flatulence.[186] Topical applications for dental pain are used in some countries, which contain the essential oil extracted from cloves, called eugenol. This oil has been applied to teeth and gums for many years, but the US Food and Drug Administration (FDA) has now reclassified eugenol — downgrading its efficacy rating, as insufficient good quality evidence has demonstrated its effectiveness for toothache. Eugenol is a pale yellow or colourless aromatic oil, also found in nutmeg, cinnamon, basil, and bay leaf.

Cobalt-Co

An element with atomic number 27 that is essential for life, but in minute quantities only. Cobalt is the central metallic element in vitamin B12, and providing we get enough B12 in our diets, we will get enough cobalt too. It is found in foods, such as fish, nuts, green leafy vegetables, and oats. The average intake for an adult is between 5 and 8 mcg per day. No Recommended Dietary Allowance has yet been established.[187]

Coenzyme Q10

Coenzyme Q10 (CoQ10) is a substance that is naturally present in the human body. Coenzyme Q and the whole family of associated compounds are known as ubiquinones, as they are so abundant in the animal kingdom. They are also found in most bacteria. Humans have high levels in the heart, liver, kidneys, and pancreas. There has been quite a lot of research into CoQ10 supplements, as some people with certain diseases appear to have lower levels of this compound, but no research so far has shown any value for cancer treatment, as is sometimes claimed. Coenzyme Q10 has, however, been shown to stimulate the immune system and to protect the heart from damage caused by one type of chemotherapy drug.[188] Only a few studies have been conducted to see whether CoQ10 could help prevent heart disease, and their results were inconclusive. Other research into the effects of CoQ10 in heart failure has also been inconclusive, but there is some evidence that CoQ10 may reduce the risk of some of the complications associated with heart surgery.[189]

Columbine- Aquilegia vulgaris

In the past, columbine (particularly yellow columbine), has been used to alleviate ulcers, but consumption is generally ill-advised, and care should also be taken when handling, as the seeds and roots may be highly toxic, containing cardiogenic toxins, which can affect the cardiovascular system. However, it does possess some astringent properties, which are sometimes harnessed in externally applied lotions.

Copper-Cu

Copper is an essential trace element with atomic number 29. Too much zinc consumption can inhibit copper absorption, and high levels of copper seem to inhibit zinc uptake too — they work in tandem somehow, one inhibiting the other.[190] By contrast, too little copper absorbed from the diet can inhibit iron uptake. Here are good examples of delicate balances between different elements at play again. We need copper for proper nervous and immune system function. It is also a vital component involved with energy production, neuropeptide (compounds that are involved in nerve transmission) activation, iron metabolism, connective tissue synthesis, and neurotransmitter synthesis. It is also a constituent of several important co-enzymes (compounds that enhance the actions of enzymes). Good sources are peanuts and pecans, seafoods (such as shellfish), liver, whole grains, beans, and lentils. Supplements containing copper, include copper gluconate, but a wide number of foods contain copper, so under normal circumstances we should get all we need from our diets. Findings show copper may play a role in preventing Alzheimer`s disease and cardiovascular disease. Below are The RDAs and ULs for copper.[191]

Recommended Dietary Allowances (RDAs)

- 0-6 months: male 200 mcg: female 200 mcg, AI (Adequate Intake)
- 7-12 months: male 200 mcg: female 200 mcg, AI
- 1-3 years: male 340 mcg: female 340 mcg
- 4-8 years: male 440 mcg: female 440 mcg
- 9-13 years: male 700 mcg: female 700 mcg
- 14-18 years: male 890 mcg: female 890 mcg; pregnancy 1,000 mcg; lactation 1,000 mcg
- 19 plus years: male 900 mcg: female 900 mcg; pregnancy 1,300 mcg; lactation 1,300 mcg

Tolerable upper limits or upper intake levels vary according to age and are shown below for copper.

Upper limits (ULs)

- 0-12 months: not possible to establish
- 1-3 years: male 1,000 mcg: female 1,000 mcg
- 4-8 years: male 3,000 mcg: female 3,000 mcg
- 9-13 years: male 5,000 mcg: female 5,000 mcg
- 14-18 years: male 8,000 mcg: female 8,000 mcg; pregnant and lactating both 8,000 mcg
- 19 years plus: male 10,000 mcg: female 10,000 mcg; pregnant and lactating both 10,000 mcg

The only sources of copper for children aged 0-12 months should come from breast milk, formula, and food.

Cranberry- Vaccinium macrocarpon, Vaccinium oxycoccos

Cranberry plants belong to a group of low growing, sometimes trailing, evergreens with small leathery leaves. The berries can be eaten or pulped into juice, and have a distinctive tart, sweet and sour flavour. The native British species is V. oxycoccus. The North American cranberry is called V. macrocarpon. Folk remedies for bladder, stomach, and liver disorders, as well as treatment for diabetes and wound healing, were common amongst the indigenous American peoples — who also used cranberries for dyeing their woven products. Today cranberry is taken as a dietary supplement and primarily used to help with urinary tract infections. Research has yielded mixed results that are often inconclusive. However, a 2012 review of 13 trials suggested certain groups, including women with recurrent urinary tract infections, children, and anyone using cranberry-containing products twice daily, might lower their risk of acquiring infections in the first place.[192]

Curcumin

Curcumin is a bright yellow product obtained from the root of turmeric, a flowering plant related to ginger, often sold as a colouring and food flavouring. It is thought, in some quarters, that the active ingredient can help with normal joint functioning, but a "cause and effect" relationship remained unproven at the time of EFSA reporting in 2017.[193] Nevertheless, later that same year, an October 2017 study, concluded that curcumin might help in the management of various oxidative and inflammatory conditions, including arthritis, anxiety, hyperlipidaemia, and metabolic syndrome.[194]

Cysteine

Cysteine is considered a semi-essential amino acid, which means that whilst it can be synthesised in the human body — on occasions demands increase, particularly in growing children or if we are unwell. This extra requirement can be derived from high-protein foods in our diets, such as eggs and poultry. It is also found in red peppers, garlic, and onions. Cysteine along with other amino acids methionine, homocysteine, and taurine contain sulphur — some of these have powerful antioxidant effects. It also helps to build hair, skin, and nails, and is vital for the synthesis of another important antioxidant compound, glutathione. Glutathione is a compound found in plants, animals, fungi, some bacteria, and archaea (a domain of single celled microorganisms that may be up to 3.5 billion years old and possibly the most ancient form of life). Glutathione is considered a major chemical factor, playing a vital role in the regulation of cell life, proliferation, and death.[195]

D

Vitamin D

Vitamin D is a fat-soluble vitamin that is best absorbed in the presence of fat, when eating a meal, or taken as a supplement.[196] It is essential for the absorption of calcium and phosphate — to keep bones, teeth, and muscles healthy. Research suggests this hormone acts as a steroid hormone and has additional wide-ranging functions, influencing the intestines, immune, cardiovascular systems, pancreas, and brain. Vitamin D is also involved in the control of cell cycles. It is believed that vitamin D insufficiency or mild deficiency is very widespread, affecting almost 50% of the population worldwide. This insufficiency is also evident throughout the European population and has been described as a pandemic, although stronger data is required for such a confident description to be used regarding Europe.[197] We need ultraviolet-B (UVB) from sunlight (vitamin D is sometimes referred to as the "sunshine vitamin"), as it induces vitamin D production in the skin, and few foods contain vitamin D in high enough quantities to satisfy our requirements. Sources include oily fish, salmon and tuna, red meat, beef liver, egg yolks, and fortified foods. So, this "pandemic" could partially be related to reduced engagement in outdoor activities and consequently less exposure to UVB. Other factors that can affect our exposure include environmental factors that reduce the absorption of sunlight through both air pollution, and different skin pigmentations — found in various populations. Darker skinned individuals absorb more UVB in the melanin of their skin than those with lighter skins, and therefore require more sun exposure to produce the same amounts of vitamin D, compared to those with less melanin. It is worth noting that wearing a sunscreen of even factor 30 can reduce vitamin D synthesis in the skin by as much as 95%. Those people with a body mass index (BMI) above 30 may have lower levels of circulating vitamin D too. This is because more is locked or stored in the fatty tissues, and as a result is less bioavailable. Additionally, vitamin D insufficiency or hypovitaminosis D is thought to be an independent risk factor associated with increased total mortality in the general population.[198] Consequently, increased levels of vitamin D supplementation have been suggested by some healthcare providers to fill any gaps. The recommended sources for this essential vitamin are either vitamin D2 (ergocalciferol) that is usually found in yeasts and some plants, including mushrooms and other plants containing endophytic fungi (fungi that live inside the plant tissue, for at least part of their life cycle, without causing apparent disease to the host plant),[199] or animal sourced vitamin D3 (cholecalciferol). The normal suggested daily amounts are around 8.5 to 10 mcg (micrograms) per day for babies, children, and adults — the suggested US figures increase as we get older (please see below). The majority of people should get enough vitamin D in the northern hemisphere between early April and the end of September. In the southern hemisphere, where seasons are reversed, people should get enough vitamin D in the southern summer. It has been found that supplementation, when necessary, has the greatest benefit on vitamin D status, if ingested during and after winter; winter officially starts on the 1st June in the southern hemisphere.[200] However, those at risk of deficiency should supplement throughout the year — with a suggestion of around 10 mcg per day.[201] Whilst it is impossible to overdose through sunlight alone, long periods of exposure to the sun`s ultraviolet rays are associated with other health risks, such as damage to the skin (increased cancer risk), eyes, and immune system. Always consult your doctor before supplementing, as some medical conditions may require lower amounts. Too much vitamin D can cause hypercalcaemia, a condition where too much calcium builds up in the blood, potentially forming deposits in the soft tissues and arteries, potentially leading to high blood pressure.[202] [203] The RDAs and ULs for vitamin D are shown below and are listed in micrograms and international units (IUs) (the biological activity of 40 IUs is equivalent to 1 mcg).[204]

Recommended Dietary Allowances (RDAs)

- 0-12 months: male 10 mcg (400 IUs): female 10 mcg (400 IUs), AI (adequate Intake)
- 1-13 years: male 15 mcg (600 IUs): female 15 mcg (600 IUs)
- 14-18 years: male 15 mcg (600 IUs): female 15 mcg (600 IUs); pregnancy 15 mcg (600 IUs); lactation 15 mcg (600 IUs)
- 19-50 years: male 15 mcg (600 IUs): female 15 mcg (600 IUs); pregnancy 15 mcg (600 IUs); lactation 15 mcg (600 IUs)
- 51-70 years: male 15 mcg (600 IUs): female 15 mcg (600 IUs)
- Greater than 70 years: male 20 mcg (800 IUs): female 20 mcg (800 IUs)

Tolerable upper limits or upper intake levels vary according to age and are shown below for vitamin D.

Upper limits (ULs)

- 0-6 months: male 25 mcg (1,000 IUs): female 25 mcg (1,000 IUs)
- 7-12 months: male 38 mcg (1,500 IUs): female 38 mcg (1,500 IUs)
- 1-3 years: male 63 mcg (2,500 IUs): female 63 mcg (2,500

- 4-8 years: male 75 mcg (3,000 IUs): female 75 mcg (3,000 IUs)
- 9-18 years: male 100 mcg (4,000 IUs): female 100 mcg (4,000 IUs); pregnant and lactating both 100 mcg (4,000 IUs)
- 19 years plus: male 100 mcg (4,000 IUs): female 100 mcg (4,000 IUs); pregnant and lactating both 100 mcg (4,000 IUs)

Dandelion Root- Taraxacum

Dandelion has been used in traditional settings for many centuries, including in Native American, traditional Chinese, and Arabic medicines. Historically, all parts of the plant were used for liver, gallbladder, and minor digestive problems. A 2017 paper showed potential for dandelion root extracts in suppressing gastric cancer cell proliferation and subsequent migration.[205] However, there is very little compelling evidence available to support mainstream medical usage. Dandelion greens contain high levels of vitamins A, C, and K, and moderate amounts of calcium, potassium, iron, and manganese.[206]

Devil`s Claw-Harpagophytum radix

The seed pods of this herb are hook shaped, hence its botanical name. A devil`s claw is a metal hook for grabbing a ship's anchor chain, resulting in its colloquial name. The hooks help with seed dispersion by animals, as the seed pods become entangled in animal fur or feathers, and are subsequently carried to new sites, often over large distances. The roots and tubers have some medicinal properties. Traditional uses included treating gout, back pain, tendonitis, heart burn, fever, and headaches. It has been used in the past as a topical application to treat both wounds and skin conditions. The active ingredient is a compound called harpagoside, which has been used for centuries by the Khosian (non-Bantu peoples) of Southern Africa to treat diverse health disorders, including diabetes, hypertension, and some blood related diseases.[207] The Committee on Herbal Medicinal Products (HMPC) concluded, in an updated assessment in 2016, that Harpagophytum radix can be used for the relief of minor joint pain, for the relief of mild digestive disorders, including bloating and flatulence, and also for the temporary loss of appetite.[208] Devil`s claw taken alone, with other ingredients, or along with non-steroidal anti-inflammatory drugs (NSAIDs) might help to decrease some osteoarthritis-related pains. Additionally, devil`s claw consumption can reduce the dose of NSAIDs required to achieve pain relief associated with osteoathritis.[209]

DHA

Docosahexaenoic acid (DHA) is an important omega-3 fatty acid important for the growth and development of the infant brain. It is also required for the maintenance of brain function in adults. Even though it is not considered essential, the body does not make appreciable amounts, so we need to get DHA from the diet or through supplementation. The full extent and consequences of dietary omega-3 fatty acid deficiency are not yet completely understood. It is believed that suboptimal intakes of ALA (Alpha-Linolenic Acid), EPA (Eicosapentaenoic acid), and DHA particularly have an association with coronary heart disease.[210] [211] Additionally, DHA is important for healthy skin and maintaining the structure of the retina. Some studies have also shown a correlation between fish consumption, rich in DHA, and the reduction in sudden death events from myocardial infarction or heart attack.[212]

D-Alpha Tocopherol

One of the eight naturally occurring forms of vitamin E. The others are beta-, gamma-, delta-tocopherol, and alpha-, beta-, gamma-, and delta-toctrienol — all with varying levels of biological activity.

E

Vitamin E

Vitamin E is a group of fat-soluble vitamins, compounds that include tocopherols and tocotrienols, as mentioned above under D-Alpha Tocopherol that are found in a wide range of foods, including soya, corn and olive oils, nuts, seeds, and wheatgerm. Vitamin E was the fifth vitamin to be discovered after conduction of animal studies in 1922, originally known as substance X, before being named as a true vitamin.[213] Vitamin E wasn`t isolated in its pure form until 1935, by Gladys Anderson Emerson, an American historian, biochemist, and nutritionist. She extracted the compounds from wheat germ oil.[214] Vitamin E helps maintain normal bone, teeth and hair, protects the lens of the eye, contributes to normal cognitive function, strengthens the immune system – the body`s natural defence system – and is a powerful antioxidant for cell protection.[215] Daily requirements, according to NHS UK, are around 4 mg for men and 3 mg for women.[216] The RDAs for this group of compounds is shown below, and we can see the US recommendations (updated 28th February 2020) appear higher than NHS UK guidance.[217]

Recommended Dietary Allowances (RDAs)

- 0-6 months: male 4 mg: female 4 mg, AI (Adequate Intake)

- 7-12 months: male 5 mg: female 5 mg, AI
- 1-3 years: male 6 mg: female 6 mg
- 4-8 years: male 7 mg: female 7 mg
- 9-13 years: male 11 mg: female 11 mg
- 14 plus years: male 15 mg: female 15 mg; pregnancy 15 mg; lactation 19 mg

Echinacea- Echinacea purpurea

Echinacea is a member of the daisy family, a genus of flowering plants with nine or ten species. The important ones used in folk medicine are Echinacea purpurea, Echinacea angustifolia, and Echinacea pallid. They are all native to North America, and were traditionally used to treat coughs, sore throats, and headaches. Echinacea is also used topically for wounds and skin problems. It is found in a wide number of food supplements, and many studies conducted into effects on the common cold have found that taking Echinacea, while you are well, may slightly reduce your chances of catching a cold. Research into certain bacteria living within the plant, itself, is ongoing, as the chemical substances in the bacteria themselves may be responsible for the beneficial effects on the human immune system.[218]

Ellagic Acid

Ellagic acid is a well-studied phytochemical, an eco-friendly phenol, with broad-spectrum antimicrobial and antioxidant properties. It can be found in a wide range of fruits and vegetables, including blackberries, raspberries, walnuts, pomegranates, and other plant foods.[219] Ellagic acid can also be extracted from the medicinal mushroom Phellinus linteus, which grows on mulberry trees. For centuries, in traditional Chinese medicine, Phellinus linteus has been consumed in combination with reishi and maitake mushrooms, and is still a popular medicinal mushroom, widely found and used in China, Korea, Japan, and some other Asian countries. It contains several bioactive compounds, including ellagic acid and caffeic acid (both natural chemicals with known antioxidant effects).[220]

Eleuthero- Eleutherococcus senticosus

Eleuthero, sometimes known as Siberian ginseng, is a species of small shrub native to Japan, northern China, Southeastern Russia, and other Northeastern Asian areas, which has been used as an immune system booster and stimulant in traditional or folk medicine settings for centuries, but only marketed as a supplement in the US, since the early 1970s. It is sometimes known as an adaptogen (a nontoxic substance, often extracted from plants that may help the body physiologically adapt to stress). It might be effective in bipolar disorder treatment. Eleuthero has been the subject of quite a lot of research, with one study showing benefits of consumption, when compared with subjects taking a combination of lithium and fluoxetine (a well-known antidepressant). The study yielded similar responses from both treatment regimens over a six-week period.[221] Additionally, it might be helpful for relieving the symptoms associated with the common cold, when used in conjunction with another herb, called andrographis, but only if taken within 72 hours of symptom onset. Eluthero might also be better than echinacea for relieving symptoms in children. When taking a product containing eleuthero, echinacea, and Malabar nut for 6 days, an improvement in the symptoms of coughing and congestion was considered better than taking a conventional drug called bromohexine — known as Kan Jang (the Swedish Herbal Institute). Other testing concluded that an extract of eleuthero appeared to decrease blood glucose levels in those with type 2 diabetes.[222] Yet another study has shown that taking eleuthero extract (Eleutheroside) seems to reduce the severity and duration of Herpes simplex 2 infections.[223] Herpes simplex 2 is a viral infection, affecting the genital region mainly. Herpes simplex 1 is the more common cold sore, often causing oral herpes infections.

EPA

Eicosapentaenoic acid is an omega-3 fatty acid that is one of the three main types — the others are ALA, already discussed under Letter A, and DHA, discussed under Letter D. In general terms EPA is thought to support the heart, immune system, and inflammatory responses. DHA is linked more to the brain, eyes, and central nervous system function. ALA is inefficiently converted into EPA and DHA, the other two omega-3 fatty acids, and at different rates — conversion to DHA is the most severely restricted.[224] On this basis it is recommended to obtain both DHA and EPA from other sources, with oily fish, krill oil, and algae oils particularly rich in these forms.

European Elder- Sambucus- nigra

The berries of this flowering tree, known as elderberries, need to be cooked prior to consumption, as they are poisonous, containing some toxic compounds known as cyanogenic glycosides. Elderberries are rich in vitamin C and are also considered moderate sources of vitamin B6 and iron. They have been used for centuries in traditional medicines, but insufficient research currently exists to establish or corroborate any of the claimed medical benefits. Sambucus nigra, the European elder, is native to Europe and parts of Asia and Africa, but also grows in the United States. The bark, leaves, flowers, fruits, and roots have been used in folk medicines since at least Anglo-Saxon times, if not before. A small number of human studies have evaluated European elder for various health conditions, with weak findings indicating that elderberry may relieve flu symptoms. Combination products containing elder flower and other herbs may be useful for sinusitis symptoms, and some research into its antioxidant capacity is still ongoing.[225]

European Mistletoe- Viscum album

Mistletoe is a type of parasitic plant, which is unable to make its own energy, so relies upon a host. It grows on several types of common tree, such as aspen, apple, oak, pine, and elm. The elm, itself, has been widely decimated, since the 1960s, by a fungal infection called Dutch elm disease. The American mistletoe belongs to the same order, Santalales, but is a different plant species (Phoradendron leucarpum). European mistletoe has been used in traditional folk medicines for years to treat seizures, headaches, and arthritis — these days it has been used to treat all types of cancer, but is currently only approved within trial settings. All parts, except for the roots, are used in extracts and supplement preparations. European mistletoe contains a toxic chemical, tyramine, found both in the berries and leaves, but in the highest levels within the leaves themselves. Serious poisonings and death have been reported in Europe, usually due to excessive concentrated herbal use, and particularly as a result of drinking mistletoe teas.[226] When injected, it is only sold in prescription drugs, which are not for mainstream use, as the US Food and Drug Administration has only approved treatment in clinical trials, and not for any medical conditions or cancers, so far, as alluded to above. To date, trials that have been completed have had major flaws, despite showing improved survival or quality of life, and cannot be relied upon due to several major weaknesses in methodology or incomplete data sets.[227] The National Center for Complementary and Integrative Health (NCCIH) in conjunction with the National Cancer Institute have completed a preliminary trial to ascertain the safety of injections using both mistletoe extracts and a particular cancer drug in patients with advanced cancer. This trial showed good tolerance for the combination therapy and thought it may be helpful in future study designs to evaluate the effectiveness of the mixture for specific cancer treatments.[228]

Evening primrose- Oenothera biennis

Evening primrose is a biennial plant, native to America, but is now found all over the world. It is sometimes known as night willowherb, King's-cure-all, and suncups. It has long been valued for its health benefits and used in traditional medicines. Evening primrose oil contains the fatty acid gamma-linolenic acid-GLA-, an omega-6 fatty acid, which has been associated with several health benefits. But only a small amount of evidence suggests it might be helpful for diabetic neuropathy.[229]

F

Fennel- Foeniculum vulgare

Fennel is a flowering plant belonging to the carrot family, providing a rich source of protein, fatty acids, dietary fibre, B vitamins, and important minerals, including calcium, iron, magnesium, and manganese. It has been used in traditional medicines for more than forty types of disorders, including relief for a range of ailments affecting the digestive, endocrine, reproductive, and respiratory systems. Extracts from the seeds are commonly used in food supplements. Apart from nutrient value, the plant contains several volatile compounds, including flavonoids and other phenolic compounds (continually under research for their health benefits). A 2014 review concluded that the compiled data from both in-vitro and in-vivo studies indicated a basis in pharmaceutical biology for the development and formulation of new drugs, using fennel extracts, for future clinical uses.[230]

Fenugreek- Trigonella foenum-graecum

This is an annual plant, whose leaves and seeds are highly valued ingredients used in Indian cuisine. The seeds contain high levels of iron and vitamins B1, B2, and B6. Historically fenugreek was used to treat a variety of health conditions, including digestive problems, and to induce childbirth, but sparse modern, good quality evidence exists to support putative health benefits. However, there is some weak research showing that fenugreek might increase milk production in lactating mothers, and some small inconclusive studies point to the lowering of blood sugars in type 2 diabetes patients.

Feverfew- Tanacetum parthenium

Feverfew is a flowering plant, a short-lived bushy perennial, belonging to the daisy family, sometimes known as bachelor's buttons; the flowers have white rays and yellow disk florets in summer.[231] Feverfew grows naturally throughout Europe, North and South America. It was traditionally prized as a herbal or folk medicine, historically used for the treatment of migraines, fevers, constipation, diarrhoea, and dizziness. The active ingredient thought to be responsible for several of these health benefits is the compound parthenolide, and along with the flowers and leaves, feverfew has been shown to have significant painkilling, anti-inflammatory, and fever reducing properties — confirming many of the folk uses.[232]

Fibre

This is the part of our diet derived from food that is not fully broken down by the digestive system, consisting of two elements — soluble and insoluble fibre. The profile of many foods is thought to contain both types, often in varying proportions and with distinctive properties.

Soluble Fibre

This fibre version dissolves in water and has fibres that once fermented are considered the prebiotic element in diets. Prebiotics are compounds that can help the growth of beneficial microorganisms in our own guts. The most common of these are fructo-oligosaccharides (FOS), galacto-oligosaccharides (GOS), and trans-galacto-oligosaccharides (TOS). Prebiotics have remarkable beneficial influences on human health, with negligible detrimental side effects.[233] Soluble fibre can be found in oats, mushrooms, barley, bran, beans, lentils, and peas. Psyllium is also a soluble, but non-fermentable fibre, which is discussed later under the Psyllium - Plantago entry. This is found in many food supplements.

Insoluble Fibre

Insoluble fibre is found in wheat bran, the cellulose from vegetables, and whole grains. This type of fibre provides bulking and does not dissolve in water. It is not digested but does facilitate the absorption of other nutrients and chemicals.[234]

A series of systematic reviews and meta-analyses examining dietary fibre and whole grains have found important health benefits, including reduced risk of death, and lower rates of both heart disease and type 2 diabetes.[235] One study over a nine-year period, examining 20,126 deaths in men and 11,330 deaths in women, found that fibre intake was associated with considerably lowered risks and lower total mortality — in both men and women — from cardiovascular, infectious, and respiratory diseases.[236]

NHS UK advice — based upon government guidelines — suggested in 2015 that we should all try to eat about 30 g of fibre per day. Caveats for children suggested, 2-5 year-olds should only need around 15 g per day, 5-11 year-olds about 20 g per day, and 11-16 year-olds around 25 g of fibre per day. This should always be part of a balanced diet, including plenty of fruit, vegetables, and starchy foods (preferably wholegrains), and where possible we should retain the skins on fruits and vegetables. NHS UK also believes most of us need to eat more fibre, and if we can, this could be associated with lowered risks of heart disease, strokes, type 2 diabetes, and bowel cancer.[237]

Fish oils

Fish oils are a rich source of omega-3 fatty acids DHA and EPA. These have been discussed under the Letters D and E.

Flaxseed & Flaxseed Oil- Linum usitatissimum

This plant belongs to the genus Linum. Flax or linseed has been cultivated in the cooler geographical areas of the world for thousands of years. It was initially used in the ancient Ayurveda and traditional Chinese medical systems to help with mental fatigue and to improve physical endurance. It is valuable both as a food and fibre crop, and Hippocrates, considered the father of medicine, recommended flax seeds to his patients over 2,000 years ago for the treatment of abdominal pains. Theophrastus, another eminent Greek scholar, successor to the famous philosopher Aristotle, advocated the use of flax mucilage (a thick viscous product) as a cough remedy. Later in the 8th century AD — Charlemagne, Charles the Great, King of the Franks — actually, passed laws requiring its consumption, as it was considered so valuable for the health of his subjects.[238] More recently, after flax was introduced to the US, the fibres were used to produce clothing. The common name for this plant is linseed and some further description can be found under the linseed entry later in the book.

Fluorine-F

An element with atomic number 9, which has a negative anion, called fluoride, can help to prevent tooth decay. Some would say it is essential. The Australians and New Zealanders, the US, and EU says it is not, but the World Health Organisation is ambivalent on the subject.[239]

Folic acid

This is a water-soluble vitamin, also known as vitamin B9, folacin or folate. Its name is derived from the Latin for leaf, as it was first isolated from spinach leaves in 1941. There are some diseases that can result in reduced absorption of this essential vitamin, such as Crohn`s disease (an inflammatory bowel disorder) — with decreased absorption leading to potential deficiency. B9 is important for prevention of neural tube defects in the early stages of human development — consequently supplements are recommended for women who are planning for pregnancy, might be pregnant, are pregnant or are breastfeeding. Folates can also contribute to good fertility through spermatogenesis.[240] Additionally, vitamin B9 is important for the treatment or prevention of folate deficiency anaemia, which is comparable to vitamin B12 anaemia — the main feature of these types of anaemia are underdeveloped red blood cells that are larger than normal. It has also been found that folate is associated with a reduction in the side effects from Methotrexate (a chemotherapy agent and immune system suppressant drug) treatment, the most common of which are nausea and vomiting. NHS UK recommends that if you are either pregnant or trying for a baby that 400 mcg of folic acid taken daily until 12 weeks of pregnancy (the end of the first trimester) can help the baby grow normally. This can be taken in tablet form with a drink, and with or without food.[241] Folate is found in a variety of foods, but only in small amounts, these include broccoli, Brussels sprouts, leafy greens, peas, chickpeas, and fortified cereals. Liver also contains vitamin B9, but should be avoided during pregnancy, as it contains high amounts of vitamin A that can cause birth defects. The full RDAs and Adequate Intakes (AIs), where appropriate, are shown below. Dietary folate equivalents (DFEs) are used for these charts, as around 85% of folic acid is estimated to be bioavailable when taken with food, whereas, in the region of 50%, of naturally occurring folates present in foods are considered bioavailable, and consequently able to enter the circulation.[242]

Recommended Dietary Allowances (RDAs)

- 0-6 months: male 65 mcg (micrograms) DFEs: female 65 mcg DFEs and AI
- 7-12 months: male 80 mcg DFEs: female 80 mcg DFEs and AI
- 1-3 years: male 150 mcg DFEs: female 150 mcg DFEs
- 4-8 years: male 200 mcg DFEs: female 200 mcg DFEs
- 9-13 years: male 300 mcg DFEs: female 300 mcg DFEs
- 14-18 years: male 400 mcg DFEs: female 400 mcg DFEs; pregnancy 600 mcg DFEs; lactation 500 mcg DFEs
- 19 plus years: male 400 mcg DFEs: female 400 mcg DFEs; pregnancy 600 mcg DFEs; lactation 500 mcg DFEs

In 1998 the Institute of Medicine (IOM) set the tolerable upper intake level (UL) at 1,000 micrograms (mcg) per day for folic acid (derived from both foods fortified with folic acid and vitamin supplementation).[243] A large number of countries have mandatory folic acid fortification programs, and the updated 2017 list of at least 84 countries includes the US, Australia, Canada, and South Africa, but not other European countries.[244] As recently as September 2021 the UK government announced that Folic acid is to be added to UK flour to help prevent spinal birth defects.[245]

Foxglove- Digitalis purpurea

Extracts of foxglove, called digitalin or digitalis, are used in medicines to increase cardiac contractility. This discovery was originally accredited to a Scottish doctor, William Withering, in 1775, when one of his patient's seeking treatment for a very bad heart condition, sourced a secret herbal remedy from a local gypsy and promptly improved. William quizzed the gypsy and discovered the plant digitalis purpura, or purple foxglove, had been used in a herbal combination taken by his patient, and the active ingredient thought responsible for the improvement was subsequently found in foxglove itself.[246] This herbaceous shrub is not for general consumption, though, as it is toxic and can cause swathes of nasty symptoms. Some species are considered deadly.

Fructooligosaccharides (FOS)

FOS (prebiotics) are naturally occurring oligosaccharides found in plants, including chicory, onion, garlic, asparagus, banana, artichoke, leeks, barley, dandelion greens, and many others. All these plants contain this prebiotic soluble dietary fibre, one property of which is to help stimulate the growth of friendly bacteria in the gut,[247] thereby improving the composition of the microbiome, as discussed in the introduction, also under sections, including, lactobacillus — mushrooms, moulds, and yeasts — and prebiotics. The microbiome or microbiota has a massive role to play in the induction, training, and function of the human immune system, which needs to maintain a symbiotic (a mutually beneficial association between different elements, e.g. humans and microbes) relationship with many microorganisms.[248] FOS have a number of other interesting and important physiological effects, such as improving mineral absorption, decreasing serum levels of cholesterol and phospholipids, with low carcinogenicity properties.[249] They are often included in food supplements for these reasons. Prebiotics should not be confused with probiotics, which contain the various strains of useful bacteria, and sometimes yeasts too. The most common groups of probiotics are Lactobacillus and Bifidobacterium, with a large range of different species that will be discussed later in the book under the probiotics entry.

G

Garcinia Cambogia- Garcinia gummi-gutta

Garcinia, also known as Malabar tamarind, is a tropical fruit that looks a bit like a pumpkin, but with a very sour taste, as it contains hydroxycitric acid. The rind of its fruit is often used to preserve food and to flavour fish curries. The seeds are rich in fat and frequently used in Indian, Indonesian, Malaysian, Sri Lankan, and Thai cuisine. In a recent 2016 animal study, hydroxycitric acid, was linked with some weight-loss benefits,[250] and may have some effect in breaking down kidney stones by directly dissolving calcium oxalate (the compound commonly found in stones).[251] However, a quality human study in 1998, concluded that Garcinia cambogia did not perform better than a placebo in producing significant weight and fat mass loss in trial participants.[252]

Garlic- Allium sativum

Garlic is a plant belonging to the onion genus with an edible bulb popular in many global cuisines — edible to humans at least, but toxic to cats and small dogs. It was originally native to north-eastern Iran and Central Asia. The largest producer today is China. Garlic was used historically for its perceived health benefits by Egyptians, Greeks, Romans, Chinese, Japanese, and Native Americans. Modern research reveals conflicting evidence about the cholesterol-lowering effects of garlic, and there is only weak evidence that it may help with high blood pressure. However, there are some studies that indicate that some groups of people who eat greater quantities of garlic may be less likely to develop certain cancers, such as stomach and colon cancers, but the dietary supplement form of garlic is not recommended by The National Cancer Institute as it does not appear to sufficiently reduce the risks of these specific cancers. Garlic appears to be safe in the quantities normally ingested in foods.[253]

Ginger- Zingiber officinale

Ginger is a tropical plant with purple-green flowers and an aromatic underground rhizome. Ginger has been used in traditional Chinese medicine and Indian Ayurvedic medicine for over 2,000 years; the dried powder was used to treat stomach aches, diarrhoea, and nausea. It is also a popular culinary ingredient as it has a pungent, piquant flavour adored by many. Ginger contains a wide variety of compounds, including manganese, magnesium, potassium, vitamin B6, and various phenolics, such as gingerol and gingerdiol. A 2017 review concluded that ginger exerted strong anti-inflammatory effects and also had anti-tumourgenic activity, thereby validating its possible nutraceutical applications.[254] Another recent systematic review found that ginger, when used as a herbal medicine, could be beneficial for, pain, nausea, and vomiting, and also helpful for metabolic syndrome — a term for a combination of diabetes, high blood pressure, and obesity. [255] Whilst some evidence exists for the relieving of pregnancy-related nausea and vomiting, it is unclear whether ginger is helpful for post-surgery nausea, motion sickness, rheumatoid arthritis, or osteoarthritis.[256]

Ginseng- Panax ginseng

Panax ginseng is also known as Asian ginseng and is native to the Far East, including China and Korea. The roots have been used in many traditional medicines for over 2,000 years. There are several types of ginsengs, including Panax quinquefolius or American ginseng, and Eleutherococcus senticosus, known as Siberian ginseng, but neither is related to true ginseng. In traditional Chinese medicine, Asian ginseng was used as a stimulant to replenish energy and revitalise. Today it can be found in many dietary supplements and is thought to improve physical stamina and concentration, stimulate the immune system, slow the aging process, and can help to relieve symptoms from numerous other disorders. Animal studies have shown some anti-obesity effects, and the ginsenoside compounds, which red ginseng contains, have also been linked with certain anticancer properties. [257] There is some evidence that suggests Asian ginseng may affect blood sugar levels and could also lower blood pressure. There have been some questions raised as to long-term safety, but very little conclusive evidence exists regarding any safety issues, or indeed, to support other health benefits.[258]

Glucomannan

Glucomannan is a natural water-soluble dietary fibre, often used in food supplements, and extracted from the roots of the elephant yam (konjac). A study from the British Journal of Nutrition on the effects of consuming gelled konjac glucomannan fibre on energy intake in healthy individuals concluded, in January 2018, that konjac may potentially introduce a new tool for body weight regulation. This occurs, effectively, through substitution with common high carbohydrate foods, such as pasta, without changing meal volume or palatability.[259] Another study concluded that glucomannans have unique functional and nutritional properties that can provide health benefits to us. In a hydrolysed form they also have prebiotic properties (stimulating the growth of friendly bacteria in the gut).[260]

Glucosamine Hydrochloride

There is an ongoing debate, with mixed findings, as to whether glucosamine, an amino acid that is produced naturally in humans, is effective in preventing progression or improving pain in large joint arthritis, and whether it can help to repair damaged hyaline cartilage. The two-year Glucosamine/Chondroitin Arthritis Intervention Trial (GAIT) concluded that use of glucosamine hydrochloride as a monotherapy was not supported – but treatment with glucosamine plus chondroitin sulphate may have benefits, with a subset of trial participants getting significant relief by using the combination therapy.[261]

Glucosamine Sulphate

As opposed to glucosamine hydrochloride, glucosamine sulphate, a naturally occurring chemical found in the fluid around joints, is rated as probably effective in providing pain relief from osteoarthritis, especially of the knees.[262] Additionally, it may slow the breakdown of joints and prevent osteoarthritis from getting worse, if taken for several years. Those taking a supplement might be less likely to need total knee replacement surgery too.[263] So, products containing glucosamine sulphate appear superior to those containing glucosamine hydrochloride, but neither appear to prevent osteoarthritis in the first place.

Golden Rod- Solidago virgaurea

This flowering herbaceous perennial belongs to the Aster family and is mostly native to North America and Mexico. This particular variety, S.virgaurea, is known as European goldenrod, and is one of a hundred or so species of the genus Solidago. The young leaves are edible, and herbal teas or infusions can be made from them. The seeds of some species have also been used in the past as a food source, particularly by Native Americans. It was traditionally used to treat painful cramping associated with menstruation, arthritis, and when topically applied, for relieving some skin conditions. Remedies based upon extracts have shown efficacy in treating infections and inflammation, preventing kidney stone formation, and are considered helpful for removal of urinary gravel.[264]

Goldenseal- Hydrastis Canadensis

This plant is native to North America, a perennial belonging to the buttercup family. It is known as yellow root or sometimes orange root, and is grown commercially, largely in the Blue Ridge Mountains of the United States. Historically, the root has been used in a traditional setting to treat skin disorders, fevers, and ulcers — by both Native Americans and European settlers. Very little research has been conducted, to date, establishing any medical benefits. However, The National Center for Complementary and Integrative Health (NCCIH) has been funding research to study how goldenseal may act against bacteria, and to find methods of developing good quality goldenseal for use in human studies.[265] Goldenseal contains berberine, an ammonium salt (Please see the berberine entry earlier in the book) found in several plant species, but only small quantities of the actual berberine compound are absorbed into the bloodstream when people ingest goldenseal orally. According to the American Cancer Society, long-term use may lead to vitamin B deficiency, hallucinations, and delirium. Also, pregnant, or breastfeeding women are advised not to use goldenseal, and it should not be given to infants at all — berberine can cause or worsen jaundice in newborn infants, which in turn can lead to brain damage in a rare condition called kernicterus.

Gotu kola- Centella asiatica

Gotu kola or Indian pennywort is used in Asian cooking, often in salads, and as a traditional medicine for treating minor wounds, but potential cardiovascular benefits and dermatological effects have limited supporting clinical data.[266]

Grape- Vitis vinifera & Vitis labrusca & Grape seed extracts

The extracts of some varieties of grape contain significant concentrations of polyphenols and flavonoids, which have proven antioxidant, antimicrobial, and antifungal effects.[267] A meta-analysis of sixteen studies has demonstrated that grape seed extracts can exert a beneficial impact on blood pressure, particularly in younger people and obese individuals.[268] Grapes themselves contain moderate amounts of vitamin K, important for blood clotting and wound healing (please see the vitamin K entry). The grape seeds and leaves also provide extracts that may help with poor circulation that can cause the legs to swell in a condition known as chronic venous insufficiency (CVI). Research has shown that taking grape seed extract or proanthocyanidins, natural polyphenols, orally for six weeks, actually decreased leg swelling.[269] A 2016 study also demonstrated the protective effects of grape seed proanthocyanidin extracts for diabetic retinopathy (DR) — a condition caused by damage to the blood vessels in the tissues at the back of the eye, within the layer known as the retina, which is sensitive to light.[270] A meta-analysis of randomised controlled trials, in 2011, found some conflicting results in humans, but still concluded that grape seed extracts may have some heart benefits, including lowering both systolic blood pressure and heart rate. The lowered heart rate may be the cause of the decreased systolic blood pressure. The extracts had no effect on lipid levels such as cholesterol, or C-reactive protein (CRP) quantities — a chemical indicator of inflammation in the arteries.[271] From 2016, The National Center for Complementary and Integrative Health (NCCIH) began supporting preliminary research into grape seed extracts and their possible beneficial effects for Alzheimer's disease sufferers, and for hereditary hemochromatosis (a condition causing high body iron levels). Some other preliminary studies support possible beneficial effects that these extracts may have in the prevention of prostate, lung, and colon cancer.[272]

Grapefruit- Citrus paradise

Grapefruit is a subtropical citrus tree, an accidental hybrid or cross between a sweet orange (C. sinensis) and a pomelo (C. maxima), originating from Barbados, with both the initial parent fruit trees hailing from Asia — probably in the seventeenth century.[273] This citrus fruit has sweet and sour flavours, with bitter notes or undertones. Nutritionally, grapefruit is a rich source of vitamin C. The fruit, oil from the peel, and extracts from the seeds are used as medicines, taken orally to support weight loss. Certain products containing sweet orange, blood orange, and grapefruit extracts seem to help decrease body weight. A 2011 study showed that preloading with grapefruit and grapefruit juice might be a good weight loss strategy, and the preload groups also experienced significantly greater benefits in their lipid profiles.[274] Some research in 2006 showed that obese candidates taking fresh grapefruit, grapefruit juice, or grapefruit capsules lost more weight than the trial placebo group over a 12-week period. Additionally, insulin resistance in tested subjects was improved by consumption of fresh grapefruit.[275] Grapefruit, however, contains a chemical, a Furanocoumarin that is present in a number of edible plants, which can interfere with the break-down of certain statin medications — so care needs to be taken.

Green tea- Camellia sinensis

Green tea has been drunk in China and Japan for many centuries and has been culturally very important in both of these countries; sometimes referred to as "the elixir of youth" in some parts of China, in the 8th Century, and considered a national obsession since its introduction by travelling merchants to the people of Japan in around the 9th Century AD.[276] Tea extracts contain flavonoids and polyphenols, which are the subjects of a great deal of in-vivo research, regarding possible health benefits. We have come across these compounds several times before, as they are found in many other plants. Green, black, and oolong teas are all derived from the same plant (Camellia sinensis), but different methods are used in their preparations. Green tea, for example, is made from lightly steaming the leaves and can also be found in liquid extracts, capsules, and tablets, and is sometimes found in topical creams applied to the skin. A small 2020 study concluded that green tea extracts improved hemodynamic and metabolic parameters, and renal function in patients with Diabetes Mellitus Type 2. Extracts also helped those suffering with chronic kidney disease.[277] Whilst considered safe across a wide range of intakes and preparations, the levels of the solid form should not supersede 338 mg of the flavanol called epigallocatechin-3-gallate (EGCG) per day, and levels in beverage form should not supersede 704 mg per day — as too much green tea consumption has been linked with liver damage.[278] One study has shown that EGCG could significantly reduce weight in women with central obesity, without any detrimental side-effects.[279] Another preclinical study showed the anti-carcinogenic properties in a prostate cancer model — when green tea extract was used in conjunction with another flavonoid called quercetin.[280] There is also evidence that green tea enhances mental alertness, but this is probably due to its caffeine content. The US Food and Drug Administration has approved a specific ointment containing green tea extracts for treating genital warts, but this is only available on prescription. There is limited evidence that both green tea and black tea may reduce some heart disease risk factors, including blood pressure and cholesterol levels.[281]

Guarana- Paullinia cupana

This climbing plant is native to the Amazon basin and is named after the Guarani or Tupi-Guaranian people of Bolivia, Paraguay, and southern Brazil.[282] The indigenous peoples at one time brewed a drink made from the seeds, which had strong stimulant effects, mainly due to their high caffeine content. A 2017 in-vitro study showed a beneficial effect on body weight control with metabolic alteration, and concluded, that together the data demonstrated the important role of guarana as a putative therapeutic agent.[283] Another 2018 study, in animals, demonstrated that guarana prevented adipose tissue accumulation and increased energy expenditure, concluding that this could contribute to a treatment for obesity. [284]

H

Hawthorn- Crataegus monogyna & Crataegus laevigata

The hawthorn is a flowering shrub, a member of the rose family, native to Europe and other temperate regions of the world. It is well suited to the ancient art form of Bonsai planting — the nurturing of miniature trees originating in ancient Chinese horticulture, and subsequently adopted by Japanese Zen Buddists over one thousand years ago. The word "Bon-sai", quite literally means planted in a container.[285] Historical use of hawthorn in folk remedies, included treatments for heart disease, digestive disorders, kidney problems, and anxiety. The fruits are called haws, are edible, and taste a little like apples. The dried fruits of Crataegus pinnatifida or Chinese hawthorn were used in traditional Chinese medicines to aid digestion in the main, but modern Western herbalists tend to use hawthorn for the treatment of heart disease. A 2010 review journal concluded, after studying data from clinical trials, that hawthorn had low or negligible side-effects, and Crataegus preparations had significant potential as useful remedies in the treatment of cardiovascular disease — probably due to the flavonoid content.[286] Hawthorn has been studied for heart failure, and one or two short-term studies have shown some possible health benefits in this area. More recent and longer-term studies, involving large cohorts in thirteen European countries, did not confirm these benefits though, and it is thought that hawthorn may detrimentally interact with some prescription drugs.[287]

Hibiscus- Hibiscus sabdariffa

Hibiscus is a flowering plant belonging to the mallow family, with well over 600 species. Other important mallows are okra, cotton, cacao, and durian. Hibiscus sabdariffa and the H. roselle species have been used traditionally as foods, in herbal drinks, in hot and cold beverages, and as flavouring agents in the food industry. As a herbal medicine, in the western folk tradition, hibiscus has been used for centuries to treat a multitude of complaints, including upset stomachs. It was used more widely — and for a larger variety of illnesses — in Indian Ayurvedic medicine, possibly for thousands of years. The Egyptians favoured the tea form to help lower body temperature, and to treat both heart and nerve ailments. More recently, sour hibiscus tea has been investigated for its possible blood pressure lowering properties. One 2015 systematic review and meta-analysis of randomized controlled trials concluding that Hibiscus sabdariffa had a significant effect in lowering both systolic and diastolic blood pressure in humans.[288]

Honey

Honey is a sweet viscous liquid made by honeybees, sourced from plant nectar, which has been researched widely and found effective for treating burns — with direct topical applications appearing to improve skin healing. A 2014 article concluded that honey had anti-infectious, anti-inflammatory, antiexudative, antioxidant, wound healing, wound debriding, and nutritional properties.[289] Honey seems to help reduce coughing spells in children aged 2 years and older and is considered at least as effective as some over-the-counter preparations.[290] There is also some conflicting research with regards to dressings and associated reduction of healing times in people with diabetic foot ulcerations. There are other uses for honey that may be effective, which include the use of eye drops containing Manuka honey (produced from the nectar of the manuka tree, Leptospermum scoparium) for dry eyes, and topical application of manuka honey products to treat rosacea – a condition that causes redness of the face. Also, it is thought that rinsing the mouth with honey seems to help the healing of mouth ulcers associated with certain chemotherapy treatments.[291] As suggested direct application of honey preparations seems to improve wound healing, with different types of honey having different properties. Honey appears to have anti-microbial, immunomodulatory, and anti-oxidant properties that can also help with reducing excessive scar tissue formation following skin injury. Honey is both safe and cost-effective.[292]

Hops- Humulus lupulus

Modern hops are derived from their wild old-world cousins, which might be over 1.5 million years old themselves. The modern hop probably emanates from Egypt, where it was originally used as a salad food; hop usage in the brewing of beer probably goes back to the Middle Ages, in the northern and eastern parts of Europe at least. The first confirmed barley brewed beers emanated from Iran (known as Persia before 1935) in the 5th century BC, but brewing with grapes, honey, hawthorns, and rice – discovered through Chinese artefacts – dates to, as long ago as, the 7th century BC.[293]

Hops, themselves, are the flowering parts of the plant. The flavours and aromas derived from them are described in multiple ways, including floral, grassy, citrus, lemony, earthy, and even spicy. They are also used in herbal medicines and other beverages. One study showed that daily supplementation with hops over a four-week period helped with the symptoms of mild depression, anxiety, and stress in young adults.[294]

Horse Chestnut- Aesculus hippocastanum

The horse chestnut tree is a familiar one to most, originally native to the Balkan Peninsula and first introduced to the UK in the late 16th century having arrived from Turkey. The horse chestnut is now planted widely across North America as an ornamental or decorative tree. Its association with horses relates to the horseshoe-shaped scars left on the twigs after the leaves fall.[295] Traditional folk remedies, made from the extracts, were used to treat joint pain, bladder and gastrointestinal ailments, fevers, and leg cramps. Modern uses are supported by numerous studies. A 2012 systematic review of 17 studies from 1976 to 2002 suggested that the extracts could, if used for a short period of time, reduce leg pain, swelling, and irritation in sufferers of chronic venous insufficiency, and might be at least as effective as wearing compression stockings.[296] Another study showed that the active ingredient aesculin, a phytochemical, could help with male fertility, but this particular Chinese study was not considered robust enough, as participants were receiving other supplements and drugs at the same time.[297]

Horsetail- Equisetum arvense

Horsetail, also known as snake grass or mare`s tail, is an invasive, firmly embedding (because of its deep roots), perennial weed that can spread quickly — covering and squeezing out less vigorous plants. It has been used as a herbal remedy for centuries. In ancient Roman and Greek times, it was used to stop bleeding, for the treatment of kidney problems, and for wound healing. One study, using the field horsetail variety, showed a diuretic effect that needed further research to elucidate the actual mechanism of action.[298]

Hyaluronic acid

Hyaluronic acid is also known as hyaluron. It is a large molecule constituent of connective, skin, and nerve tissues, as well as the eyes. It keeps tissues well lubricated, contributing to cell number increases and movement. In its high molecular form, it can be injected into knees to treat osteoarthritis.[299]

I

Iodine-I

Iodine, atomic number 53, is an essential chemical element which helps to make thyroid hormone. The incorporation of iodine into growth regulating hormones, thyroxine, and triiodothyronine, occurs in the thyroid gland — with these hormones playing vital roles in the regulation of metabolic rate, heart and digestive functions, muscle control, brain development, and the maintenance of good bone structure. Adults require around 0.14 mg per day. Good sources include marine products, such as sea fish and shellfish. To access enough iodine from plant foods, such as cereals and grains, requires the presence of sufficient iodine in the soil, so inland areas where virtually no marine foods are eaten tend to result in deficiencies, possibly leading to hypothyroidism — an underactive thyroid gland. As a consequence, the thyroid gland does not produce enough hormones. If supplements are required, taking 0.5 mg (500 mcg) or less per day is unlikely to cause any harm.[300] The full RDA and Adequate Intake (AI) figures for iodine are shown below.[301]

Recommended Dietary Allowances (RDAs)

- 0-6 months: male 110 mcg: female 110 mcg, AI
- 7-12 months: male 130 mcg: female 130 mcg, AI
- 1-3 years: male 90 mcg: female 90 mcg

- 4-8 years: male 90 mcg: female 90 mcg
- 9-13 years: male 120 mcg: female 120 mcg
- 14-18 years: male 150 mcg: female 150 mcg; pregnancy 220 mcg; lactation 290 mcg
- 19 plus years: male 150 mcg: female 150 mcg; pregnancy 220 mcg; lactation 290 mcg

Inulin

Inulin is a type of dietary fibre found in a wide range of plants, but the form most often used in medicines is the starchy substance derived from chicory roots. When taken daily, inulin is associated with increasing stool frequency and maintaining normal defaecation.[302] Inulin is a fructan (a fruit sugar polymer), which is found in about 12% of plants, including agave, garlic, asparagus, wheat, barley, and Jerusalem artichokes. Fructans contain polysaccharides (long-chain compounds) that serve as short-term energy stores in plants, usually located within the stems of grass species, and these allow the plants to withstand sub-zero temperatures. In the food industry fructans are included as dietary fibre because of their prebiotic properties. Prebiotics are those compounds that help promote the growth of beneficial bacteria in our gastrointestinal system (Please see the prebiotics entry).[303]

Iron-Fe

Iron is one of the most abundant elements in the universe, with atomic number 26, which is essential for a wide array of human metabolic processes. These include DNA synthesis, oxygen transportation, and electron transport. However, because iron forms free radicals in the human body, its concentration needs to be tightly regulated, as excessive amounts may lead to tissue damage.[304] Homeostatic regulation — achieving the correct balance — is vital as too much iron, specifically, can increase the risk of neurodegenerative diseases, and too little makes us more susceptible to anaemia. Actual iron absorption from the diet can be at fairly low levels, sometimes as low as 2%, depending on the specific source. There are two forms of dietary iron, heme iron and non-heme iron. Heme iron comes from animal sources and is highly bioavailable (15%-35%), with other dietary factors having little effect on its absorption, whereas non-heme iron is derived from plants and is not absorbed as well, so has much lower bioavailability (2%-20%). This can be strongly modified by the presence of other foods.[305] Fortunately we tend to eat enough quantity of the foods containing non-heme iron, which to a large extent balances its lower bioavailability. Good sources of both forms of iron include liver (to be avoided in pregnancy), meat, beans, nuts, brown rice, soy-bean flour, and green leafy vegetables. NHS UK states the requirements for men over 18 and women over 50 years of age should be around 8.7 mg per day. Women between the ages of around 19 and 50 are advised to increase this to 14.8 mg per day, due to menstrual loss. The RDAs and Adequate Intake (0-6 months) for iron are shown below for non-vegetarians. The RDAs suggested for vegetarians are 1.8 times higher than for those individuals who eat meat.[306]

Recommended Dietary Allowances (RDAs)

- 0-6 months: male 0.27 mg: female 0.27 mg, Adequate Intake (AI)
- 7-12 months: male 11 mg: female 11 mg
- 1-3 years: male 7 mg: female 7 mg
- 4-8 years: male 10 mg: female 10 mg
- 9-13 years: male 8 mg: female 8 mg
- 14-18 years: male 11 mg: female 15 mg; pregnancy 27 mg; lactation 10 mg
- 19-50 years: male 8 mg: female 18 mg; pregnancy 27 mg; lactation 9 mg
- 51 years plus: male 8 mg: female 8 mg

J

Juniper- Juniperus osteosperma

There are many living species of Juniper trees and the berries have been used in traditional medicines for centuries, particularly amongst several tribes of the Americas. The ash from burnt trees was collected by the Navajo, Native American peoples of the Southwestern US, and stirred into traditional dishes, as it was generally considered good for overall health. We now know the ash is high in calcium, an essential mineral for helping build strong bones and teeth, regulating muscle contractions, and assisting with the normal clotting of blood. Juniper berries may have some side-effects in pregnant and breastfeeding women but are considered generally safe in the US. The essential oils that can be extracted from the berries of various species of juniper contain a wide variety of terpenoids and aromatic compounds. One species, J oxycedrus, provides a tar extract with a sesquiterpene compound known as cadinene; these oils are often found in cosmetic and hair products.[307] Emerging health benefits may relate to compounds that have previously been shown to have antimicrobial, anti-inflammatory, and antioxidant effects, but there remains limited research to show benefits for specific health conditions, and juniper supplements, themselves, are considered unsafe to use if pregnant or trying to become pregnant. They are best avoided when breastfeeding too.[308] The berry is often used in condiments, and as a flavouring ingredient in gin and other bitter products.

K

Vitamin K

Vitamin K is not one vitamin in fact, but a group of fat-soluble vitamins. These compounds include phylloquinone (vitamin K1) and a series of menaquinones (vitamin K2), amongst others. Vitamin K1 is the main dietary form, mostly found in green leafy vegetables, including kale, broccoli, and spinach. Vitamin K2 compounds are predominantly of bacterial origin and found in animal based and fermented foods. The bacteria in our own guts produce vitamin K2, with one particular compound of K2 derived from K1 itself.[309] Vitamin K is required for bone metabolism and blood clotting. It is therefore integral to good wound healing. The precise relationship of vitamin K with the dependant coagulation factor prothrombin, part of the blood clotting process, was not discovered until as recently as 1974.[310][311][312] Apart from green leafy vegetables, vitamin K1 is found in vegetable oils and cereal grains, with meat and dairy foods only containing small amounts. Vitamin K is rapidly metabolised in the human body, although some excess vitamin K can be stored in the liver; it has generally low blood levels and tissue stores when compared to other fat-soluble vitamins.[313]

Daily requirement

Insufficient data exists to establish an Estimated Average

Requirement (EAR) for vitamin K. NHS UK states, however, that adults require about 1 microgram (mcg) per day for each kilogram of their body weight. So, if I told you my body weight, you could calculate my daily requirement, and advise me appropriately. NHS UK also states that 1 mg or less, taken daily in supplementary form, is unlikely to cause harm.[314] Adequate intakes (AIs) for vitamin K that are not based upon NHS UK estimations, using body weight, are shown below.[315]

Adequate Intakes (AIs)

- Birth to 6 months: male 2.0 mcg: female 2.0 mcg
- 7-12 months: male 2.5 mcg: female 2.5 mcg
- 1-3 years: male 30 mcg: female 30 mcg
- 4-8 years: male 55 mcg: female 55 mcg
- 9-13 years: male 60 mcg: female 60 mcg
- 14-18 years: male 75 mcg: female 75 mcg; pregnancy 75 mcg; lactation 75 mcg
- 19 plus years: male 120 mcg: female 90 mcg; pregnancy 90 mcg; lactation 90 mcg

Kale- Brassica oleracea

Kale is a type of cabbage with edible leaves, which is a nutrient dense food containing a large array of vitamins, with particularly high levels of vitamins C and K, as well as a host of minerals, including manganese, calcium, iron, phosphorus, and magnesium. Sabellian kale is known to have been cultivated up to 4,000 years ago both in Asia Minor and the eastern Mediterranean — it was also widely consumed during the Middle Ages in Western Europe, considered the predecessor of modern kale. Kale cultivation was encouraged during World War II as part of the "Dig for Victory" campaign because of its wide nutrient content, and since 2010 Kale sprouts, known as kalettes (crosses between kale and Brussels sprouts), have become extremely popular — sometimes used to compliment other ingredients in food supplements, as they are also highly nutritious.

Kava- Piper methysticum

Kava is a member of the pepper family, which is native to the islands of the South Pacific and has been used traditionally by Pacific islanders in ceremonies to bring about a state of relaxation at many local gatherings — maybe, by engendering soporific effects. The roots are used today, as a dietary supplement, to help with symptoms of anxiety. Whilst there is evidence that kava can reduce anxiety slightly, the link between some kava compounds and an increased risk of severe liver disease is considered a major drawback.[316]

Kelp- laminaria

Kelps are types of large brown seaweeds. Some kelp species can grow to nearly 50 metres long and are often part of large kelp forests that range along about 25% of the world's coastlines. These are important habitats for a variety of invertebrates, fish, marine mammals, and birds.[317] The extracts are rich in the essential element iodine (please see the iodine entry) and are therefore important for thyroxine (T4) and triiodothyronine (T3) hormone production. These compounds help to support the skin, nervous system, and are involved with energy regulation. Raw sea kelps also contain vitamins B1, B2, B6, C, E, and K, as well as minerals, zinc, magnesium, iron, potassium, manganese, sodium, phosphorus, and calcium. Kelps also contain alginates, which are viscous compounds used in some preparations for treating GERD (gastroesophageal reflux disease).[318]

Kidney bean white- Phaseolus vulgaris

The white kidney bean is a member of the legume family

native to Middle America, with many familiar bean cultivars and varieties. They are good sources of nutrition, containing protein, excellent fibre volume and often the essential mineral potassium. These white beans are fat-free, sodium-free, and cholesterol-free, "three frees for the price of one"! However, they do contain the toxin phytohaemagglutinin, a carbohydrate binding protein present in many bean varieties, especially red kidney beans, which is only deactivated by a minimum of 10 minutes cooking at 100 degrees Celsius; some advocate even longer.[319] Several studies have shown that extracts from white kidney beans could be beneficial in reducing body weight. One study, in-particular, has shown that a daily dietary intake of circa 2,400 mg, by obese subjects, was more effective than a placebo for reducing both body weight and body fat mass over a short time period. The thought is that this probably works through inhibiting alpha-amylase, the enzyme responsible for carbohydrate breakdown.[320]

Krill oil- Euphasia superb

Antarctic krill are a rich source of phospholipid derived fatty acids and omega-3 fatty acids, which have many health benefits, discussed earlier under the ALA, EPA, and DHA entries. Krill oil is therefore a good alternative to fish oil supplements, with well-documented potential cardiovascular benefits. Patients must consume the lower dose of 1 g of both EPA and DHA for cardiac protection, or a higher dose of between 2 g and 4 g for triglyceride (a type of fat found in the bloodstream) reduction, important for cholesterol control. The higher dose tends to need supplementation, but the lower dose can be derived from dietary fish alone.[321]

L

L-Glutamine

Glutamine is the most abundant freely circulating amino acid, one of the building blocks for proteins. Whilst glutamine is classified as a non-essential amino acid, in certain disease conditions it works as an essential amino acid, working to boost immunity. Glutamine can support muscle glycogen replenishment following exhaustive exercise, supports a healthy digestive system, and also contributes to the strengthening of natural defences. Glutamine contributes to the healthy function of the nervous system and brain. As a precursor of GABA (g-amino butyric acid) and other compounds, glutamine supports concentration and mental performance under situations of mental or physical exertion, and in the elderly, it helps to maintain working memory. Extra dietary or supplement forms help to restore plasma glutamine levels after metabolic stress. It also contributes to gut protein synthesis, helping to decrease permeability of gut cells, and assists the replenishment of carbohydrate stores in both muscles and the liver. The list of benefits is long, also including an association with improvements in intestinal water and electrolyte absorption. So, glutamine is vital for repair, recovery, supporting glucose homeostasis during and after exercise, and for our natural defences (the immune system), by helping with the rapid renewal of immune cells, such as lymphocytes. [322] Dietary sources include protein rich foods, including beef, chicken, dairy-products, and eggs. Vegetables like beans, cabbage, spinach, carrots, celery, kale, and fermented foods, for example miso, are also important sources of L-glutamine. You may have seen L-theanine in some supplements, and this is an amino acid analogue (a compound having a similar structure to that of another compound) of glutamine itself.

L-Tyrosine

Tyrosine is another non-essential amino acid involved in protein synthesis. It is also found in protein rich foods, and in conjunction with phenylalanine, an essential amino acid from which tyrosine can be synthesised, has a recommended daily allowance of around 25 mg per kilogram of body weight.[323]

Lactobacillus

Lactobacillus is an important group of gut friendly bacteria, vital constituents of our microbiome, which convert sugars to lactic acid. This large genus includes the common varieties, L. casei, L.rhamnosus, L. acidophilus, and L.bulgaricus. They are considered one of the most common types of probiotics (please see the probiotic entry), and can be found in fermented foods, yogurts, and supplements. They have a symbiotic relationship with the human body; we feed them, and they protect us from pathogens.[324] Lactobacillus is also an important inhibitor of the fungal pathogen candida albicans.[325] Candida is opportunistic and becomes pathogenic under certain conditions, particularly in immuno-compromised individuals.[326] Lactobacillus might be effective for reducing stomach pain in children, when taken in the short-term. This group of bacteria ingested in the two billion strength form can improve the quality of life for people with grass pollen allergies and hay fever. When taken in the ten billion strength form, lactobacillus seems to help with itchy eye symptoms too. Taking probiotics containing lactobacillus can help prevent diarrhoea caused by antibiotic treatment, in both adults and children. A fair amount of research has shown that lactobacillus products can both prevent and reduce the symptoms of eczema, also known as atopic dermatitis. The list of possible benefits is quite extensive, including prevention of allergic reactions, and helping to prevent diabetes in mothers over 35 years of age — if taken from the beginning of the second trimester. Lactobacillus can lower total cholesterol, particularly when taken with other mainstream drugs and can also reduce digestive tract infections from bacteria, such as Helicobacter pylori. In women, it has been linked with a reduction in tenderness and swelling in the joints associated with rheumatoid arthritis and can even help with increasing remission periods for those suffering with irritable bowel syndrome (IBS), or ulcerative colitis.[327]

Lady`s Mantle- Alchemilla vulgaris

This plant is a herbaceous perennial, native to the cooler climes of Europe and Greenland. The name Alchemilla is derived from the word alchemy, as it was once thought to have magical qualities. One variety, A.mollis, has been cultivated for its ornamental value since the cultivar was first imported from southern Europe in the 19th century. Another variety, A.erythropoda, only grows naturally in the Carpathian Mountains (the second longest mountain system in Europe, covering an area of around 210,000 km^2) and the Balkans — this plant variety is also valued, as an attractive ornamental plant, by gardeners worldwide.

A.vulgaris, itself, has been used as a traditional folk medicine to treat gynaecological disorders and to alleviate symptoms from a wide range of conditions, most often brewed and consumed in tea form. Recent chemical profiling of extracts has found 26 phenolic compounds possessing good potential for various pharmaceutical applications that need further investigation.[328]

Lavender- Lavandula angustifolia and spica

This is a flowering plant belonging to the mint family. It is sometimes known as English lavender, common lavender, or French lavender. It was originally native to what was called the Old-World.[329] The essential oils that are commonly extracted and have distinctive earthy floral scents contain numerous phytochemicals; compounds that help plants defend themselves from competitors, predators, or pathogens. The oils may have some medicinal properties in humans, and extracts are often used in topical balms and perfumes. Traditionally lavender was used as a painkiller, antidepressant, an antispasmodic to relieve gastrointestinal problems, and was also thought to possess some antimicrobial properties — maybe this is one of the reasons ancient Egyptians used lavender in the ancient process of Egyptian mummification (the embalming process that delays changes to the body following death, to forestall decomposition, to some extent). The Romans used lavender oils in soaps, for cooking, bathing, and scenting the air, often transporting it with them on their travels throughout the Roman Empire.[330] The name itself is derived from the Latin verb "lavare", which means, "to wash". Extracts have sometimes been used to treat acne and headaches, and inhaling lavender vapour seems to help people get to sleep by reducing agitation associated with dementia. Most trials, however, have been considered of poor quality, with inconsistent results.[331] The results of a 1998 study thought that a combination of the herbs thyme, cedarwood, rosemary, and lavender, in oil form, might help prevent hair loss from a condition known as alopecia areata. This study also showed aromatherapy usage to be a safe and effective treatment.[332]

Linoleic acid

Linoleic acid (LA) is the most common polyunsaturated omega-6 fatty acid (please see the omega-6 fatty acid entry), which can be converted into longer omega-6 fatty acids, such as arachidonic acid. It is vital for a healthy life and is thus considered an essential compound. We tend to get enough from a balanced diet, as it is found in abundance in nuts, sesame seeds, sunflower, evening primrose, poppy seed oils, and soybeans.

Linseed oil- Linum usitatissimum

This oil is extracted from the dried ripened seeds of the flax plant — the edible form is known as flaxseed oil. The oil can be used for prolonging cricket bats and as a constituent of putty, a glazing compound, but we are interested in its nutritional value, as a common dietary supplement. Linseed contains between 57 and 71 per cent of the polyunsaturated fats ALA and linoleic acid, already discussed under the omega-3 and omega-6 fatty acids sections within this book.[333]

Liquorice- Glycyrrhiza galbra

The root of this native Mediterranean plant has been used in traditional remedies for thousands of years. It largely grows in Greece, Turkey, and Asia — these days it is most frequently found in various food and confectionery items. It was used centuries ago for treating stomach inflammation and upper respiratory tract problems. However, care needs to be taken as the saponin compound it contains, glycyrrhizic acid (GZA), has toxic properties when consumed in large quantities. Some individuals with heart or kidney problems may be more susceptible to GZA intake, but generally, a normal healthy person can consume 10 mg of GZA per day.[334] Modern studies do not support uses for any specific health conditions, and one article concerning a Finnish study of mothers and their young children suggested that eating too much liquorice during pregnancy could cause problems with brain development in the growing foetus, and future cognitive abilities in the developing offspring.[335]

Lithium-Li

This element, with atomic number 3, is predominantly found in grains and vegetables. One pilot study found that within some geographical areas, lithium could be found in drinking water in significant amounts, and this has been linked to a reduction in suicides amongst men. Consequently, it would be sensible, or one should say vitally important, for evaluation of specific lithium levels in local drinking waters to be assessed at all regional levels.[336] Another 2017 Danish study linked low lithium exposure to the prevalence of dementia in a large cohort, and very similar patterns were found with sufferers of both Alzheimer`s disease and vascular dementia. [337] Lithium is an important element for foetal development and is thought to be correlated with certain growth and transforming factors, influencing the functions of some vitamins, hormones, and enzymes.[338] Suggested intakes are estimated to be around 1,000 micrograms per day for a 70 KG adult, but the beneficial daily sweet spot is still under debate.[339] Currently there is no Recommended Dietary Allowance for lithium.

Lovage- Levisticum officinale

Lovage has been cultivated in Europe for centuries, often used in the 14th century to ease pain and help with digestion. This tall perennial herb is a relative of parsley, and originally hails from Greece; its flavour and smell is often compared to a fusion of parsley and celery. Apart from the leaves, the roots are eaten as a vegetable, and the seeds are used for spicing.[340] Lovage is now studied for its potential anti-inflammatory properties, due to the presence of various phenolic compounds, including apterin and rutin, which are both believed to act as antioxidants.[341]

Lychee-Litchi chinensis

Lychee is a tree, native to China, belonging to the soapberry family. It bears Vitamin C rich fruits, and contains moderate quantities of polyphenols, known for their antioxidant benefits, as we have previously seen. The seeds, however, contain a toxic compound called Methylene cyclopropyl acetic acid (MCPA), which is also produced in chemical reactions following ingestion of the rare amino acid hypoglycin (related to the common amino acid lysine). Hypoglycin is found in other soapberry varieties, including the unripe ackee fruit from Africa. One animal study in 1962 found this toxin could cause low blood sugars — or hypoglycaemia as it is medically known.[342]

M

Maca- Lepidium meyenii

Maca or Peruvian ginseng is mainly grown for consumption of its roots. Most of the harvested maca is dried and then powdered, and in this form, the hypocotyls, the parts just above the roots, can be stored for several years. It has a particular taste that is not loved by all, often described as earthy, nutty, and malt-like. It is thought to have several health benefits, though, with two trials in healthy men showing positive effects on improving semen quality.[343] It is acknowledged that more rigorous research is required to strengthen the systematic review conclusions with respect to all health claims.

Magnesium-Mg

Magnesium is a chemical element, with atomic number 12, which is essential for humans. Good sources of dietary magnesium are nuts, green leafy vegetables, brown rice and wholegrains, fish, meat, and dairy foods. In the human body over 300 reactions are dependent upon magnesium, including normal nerve transmission, muscle function, with a requirement for a healthy immune system — both our innate and acquired immune responses.[344] Magnesium helps to keep the heartbeat steady, contributes to bone strength, and influences blood glucose levels. On a daily basis our dietary requirement, according to NHS UK, is 300 mg for men and 270 mg for women, but at different ages and life circumstances, we need varying amounts, with 400 mg or less per day in supplementation form considered safe.[345] The full RDAs and ULs for magnesium are shown below.[346]

Recommended Dietary Allowances (RDAs)

- 0-6 months: male 30 mg: female 30 mg, Adequate Intake (AI)
- 7-12 months: male 75 mg: female 75 mg, Adequate Intake (AI)
- 1-3 years: male 80 mg: female 80 mg
- 4-8 years: male 130 mg: female 130 mg
- 9-13 years: male 240 mg: female 240 mg
- 14-18 years: male 410 mg: female 360 mg; pregnancy 400 mg; lactation 360 mg
- 19-30 years: male 400 mg: female 310 mg; pregnancy 350 mg; lactation 310 mg
- 31-50 years: male 420 mg: female 320 mg; pregnancy 360 mg; lactation 320 mg
- 51 years plus: male 420 mg: female 320 mg

Tolerable upper limits or upper intake levels vary according to age and are shown below for magnesium.

Upper limits (ULs)

- 0-12 months: not possible to establish.
- 1-3 years: male 65 mg: female 65 mg
- 4-8 years: male 110 mg: female 110 mg
- 9-18 years: male 350 mg: female 350 mg; pregnant and lactating both 350 mg
- 19 years plus: male 350 mg: female 350 mg; pregnant and lactating both 350 mg

Manganese-Mn

This is a chemical element with atomic number 25 that has various functions, including the activation of enzymes — proteins which breakdown foods in the human body. One of these important enzymes is manganese superoxide dismutase, which helps to maintain mitochondrial and cell membranes by breaking down reactive oxygen species (ROS). It is considered the chief ROS scavenging enzyme in the cell, and sometimes referred to as the "Guardian of the Powerhouse".[347] Manganese is also involved with normal growth and development processes,[348] is essential for blood clotting and haemostasis, working in close conjunction with vitamin K. Manganese is distributed widely in bone, the liver, pancreas, kidneys, and brain. A wide variety of foods contain manganese, including whole grains, mussels, clams, nuts, soybeans, leafy vegetables, coffee, tea, and black pepper. How absorption of manganese works is not clearly understood, but it is known that whilst only small amounts are utilised from the diet, efficiency increases with low intakes and decreases with high dietary intakes; an example of a negative feedback system in operation, which effectively reduces large fluctuations. The Adequate Intakes for manganese are shown below.[349]

Adequate Intakes (AIs)

- 0-6 months: male 0.003 mg: female 0.003 mg, Adequate Intake (AI)
- 7-12 months: male 0.6 mg: female 0.6 mg
- 1-3 years: male 1.2 mg: female 1.2 mg
- 4-8 years: male 1.5 mg: female 1.5 mg
- 9-13 years: male 1.9 mg: female 1.6 mg
- 14-18 years: male 2.2 mg: female 1.6 mg; pregnancy 2.0 mg; lactation 2.6 mg
- 19-50 years: male 2.3 mg: female 1.8 mg; pregnancy 2.0 mg; lactation 2.6 mg

- 51 years plus: male 2.3 mg: female 1.8 mg

Tolerable upper limits or upper intake levels vary according to age and are shown below for manganese.

Upper limits (ULs)

- 0-12 months: not possible to establish.
- 1-3 years: male 2 mg: female 2 mg
- 4-8 years: male 3 mg: female 3 mg
- 9-13 years: male 6 mg: female 6 mg
- 14-18 years: male 9 mg: female 9 mg; pregnant and lactating both 9 mg
- 19 years plus: male 11 mg: female 11 mg; pregnant and lactating both 11 mg

Mangosteen- Garcinia mangostana

The mangosteen is a tropical evergreen tree with edible fruit containing moderate nutritional value only. Knowledge regarding this plant is connected to the discovery of Saccharomyces boulardii, a tropical yeast and probiotic, by a French scientist, Henri Boulard, in the early part of the 20th century. This occurred whilst he was observing the indigenous people of Southeast Asia chewing the skins of lychees and mangosteens. They were desperately attempting to treat diarrhoea during a nasty cholera outbreak.[350] Some research has shown a possible benefit in the treatment of serious gum disease, and another scholarly article suggests that a herbal blend of Sphaeranthus indicus, colloquially known as the East Indian globe thistle, and Garcinia mangostana, appear to be both well-tolerated and an effective combination of ingredients for weight management in obese and overweight people.[351]

Marine Collagen

Marine collagen is often used as a substitute for mammalian collagen, having a wide range of applications in the food, pharmaceutical, and biomedical industries. It is used for cartilage repair and arthritis treatment, corneal treatment, and has dental applications too. In the food industry marine collagen supplements can help to maintain skin, hair, nails, and body tissues in general. Marine collagen is ubiquitous — good quality sources include the Japanese sturgeon, bighead carp, and seer fish,[352] but most feel we should derive this important protein from the most sustainable of sources, such as wild-caught North Atlantic fish, which includes pollock, haddock, and cod. However, we need to be aware of the continuing levels of persistent organic pollutants (POPs) in our oceans, despite some efforts to reduce contaminant quantities in the marine environment over several decades.[353]

Maritime Pine- Pinus pinaster Aiton

This tree grows in countries along the Mediterranean Sea. Extracts from pine nuts of the French maritime pine contain compounds used in a trademarked product called Pycnogenol. Similjjar compounds can be extracted from peanut skin, grape seed, and witch hazel bark — these have some interesting pharmacological properties. They contain polyphenols, compounds, which appear to exert long-lasting and positive effects on patients with mild osteoarthritis, by both enhancing mobility and relieving pain.[354] A systematic review conducted in 2018, also concluded that pycnogenol supplementation may have an important role to play in the prevention of cardiovascular diseases, through improving levels of HDL — the helpful cholesterol.[355] Some research shows extracts can reduce allergy symptoms caused by birch trees, if taken at the start of the season, and when taken with other asthma medications pine extracts could also be effective in decreasing asthma symptoms — this could reduce the usage of rescue inhalers. Other possible benefits, backed up by scientific evidence, include improving mental function in adults of all ages, the slowing or prevention of worsening retinal disease caused by diabetes, atherosclerosis, and other diseases — if taken over a two-month period. Additionally, extracts also appeared to improve eyesight.[356]

Mediterranean Saltbush- Atriplex halimus

The Mediterranean saltbush, also known as the sea orache, has been shown to have significant hypoglycaemic properties. Native to Europe and Northern Africa, this plant may play a role as a factor in glucose-homeostasis regulation (maintaining a stable sugar equilibrium). Both in-vitro and in-vivo evaluations of a mixture of dry extracts from the leaves of the Juglans regia (Walnut), Olea europea (Olive), Urtica dioica (Common nettle), and Atriplex halimus (Saltbush) were evaluated using various test systems, and it was found that herbal combinations of the four plants seemed to act synergistically (in a cooperative manner), but differently, to regulate glucose-homeostasis.[357]

Milk Thistle- Silybum marianum

This plant is native to Southern Europe and areas from Southern Russia to Asia, but is also found globally, now growing in North America, South America, and South Australia. It has purple flowers and pale-green leaves, which are splashed with white, hence its colloquial name. Silymarin is the main compound thought to have historical medical benefits for treatment of liver disorders and gallbladder problems, but results from modern, much more rigorous trials have been mixed. One 2008 study showed some benefits in patients who took silymarin — they experienced fewer and milder symptoms of liver disease. However, another 2012 trial concluded that silymarin was no better than a placebo for the treatment of chronic hepatitis C.[358] Milk thistle does, however, appear to stimulate prolactin, a hormone secreted from the pituitary gland. This helps females to produce milk, which is possibly due to a particular oestrogenic activity of the active compound.[359]

Molybdenum

Molybdenum is an element with atomic number 42, which is an essential constituent of just four enzymes in the human body, all with vital functions.[360] These were discovered in the 1950s and are involved in the regulation of nitrogen, sulphur, and carbon within the human body.[361] Deficiency has been linked to increased rates of oesophageal cancers in diverse geographical regions from northern China through to Iran.[362] We tend to get sufficient quantities from our diets, depending on the soil quality, and molybdenum is found in a wide range of foods, including nuts, oats, peas, leafy vegetables, and tinned vegetables. The UK daily amounts required are estimated to be around 0.075 mg (75 mcg) for men and 0.06 mg (60 mcg) for women, between the ages of 19 and 64. Regulation of molybdenum levels occurs in the kidneys, although it is also stored as a cofactor in the liver, kidney, adrenal glands, and bones. The full US RDAs for molybdenum are shown below.[363]

Recommended Dietary Allowances (RDAs)

- Birth to 6 months: male 2.0 mcg (micrograms): female 2.0 mcg: These Adequate Intakes are based on mean molybdenum intakes for infants fed on primarily human milk
- 7-12 months: male 3 mcg: female 3 mcg: AI based on mean molybdenum intakes for infants fed on primarily human milk
- 1-3 years: male 17 mcg: female 17 mcg
- 4-8 years: male 22 mcg: female 22 mcg

- 9-13 years: male 34 mcg: female 34 mcg
- 14-18 years: male 43 mcg: female 43 mcg; pregnancy 50 mcg; lactation 50 mcg
- 19 plus years: male 45 mcg; female 45 mcg; pregnancy 50 mcg; lactation 50 mcg

Tolerable upper limits or upper intake levels vary according to age and are shown below for molybdenum.

Upper limits (ULs)

- 0-12 months: not possible to establish
- 1-3 years: male 300 mcg: female 300 mcg
- 4-8 years: male 600 mcg: female 600 mcg
- 9-13 years: male 1,100 mcg: female 1,100 mcg
- 14-18 years: male 1,700 mcg: female 1,700 mcg; pregnant and lactating both 1,700 mg
- 19 years plus: male 2,000 mcg: female 2,000 mcg; pregnant and lactating both 2,000 mcg

The only sources of molybdenum for children aged 0-12 months should come from breast milk, formula, and food.

Montmorency cherry- Prunus cerasus

This tree is a hybrid of the sweet cherry and dwarf cherry, producing a sour cherry fruit, valued for its antioxidant, anti-inflammatory, and vasoactive (affecting the diameter of blood vessels) properties. Research has shown an improvement in exercise performance after just one week of supplementation,[364] and improved vascular function in overweight, middle-aged men, after 4 weeks of Montmorency cherry powder supplementation.[365] Some reports have also indicated benefits of consuming cherries for arthritis, lowering the risk of gout attacks or flare-ups, diabetes, the regulation of cholesterol levels, improving sleep quality, cognitive function, and improving general disposition. The only problem is a large number of cherries need to be consumed daily to engender most of these benefits; some think around 45-270 per day.[366] Turkey, Russia, Poland, and Ukraine are the biggest cherry producers according to The Food and Agriculture Organization of the United Nations (FAO).

Moringa oleifera

Moringa is a large tree, also known as the drumstick tree, which is native to the Indian subcontinent, but grown in both the tropics and subtropics too. It has nutritious leaves and roots that taste pungent and bitter, a bit like horseradish. The leaves are the most nutritious part of the tree, rich in several B vitamins, particularly vitamin B6, but also containing vitamin C, provitamin A, vitamin K, manganese, magnesium, and protein.[367] Apart from the leaves and roots, the immature seed pods, flowers, mature seeds, and pressed oils are also edible — maybe this is the reason some call moringa a superfood? The oils resist oxidation as they contain up to 8.6% behenic acid, an important constituent of the pressed seeds, discovered in 1848 — giving moringa oil a long storage life.[368]

MSM- Methylsulfonylmethane

MSM is used as a dietary supplement and has attracted a host of health claims over the years, some of which have been researched better than others. Some studies into possible treatments for oxidative stress and osteoarthritis (OA) have suggested some benefits. In fact, one small pilot trial, with 50 men and women, demonstrated a reduction in pain symptoms from OA, and also an improvement in physical function over a twelve-week period, and without any major adverse events.[369] Another fully fledged study conducted in 2004, included 118 patients with OA, showed significant improvement in reducing pain, inflammation, and swelling, when MSM was used in conjunction with glucosamine.[370] The Indian researchers found a reduced time to benefit, if both compounds were used together, as opposed to just taking the glucosamine, and this represents another good example of two compounds working together in synergy. A more recent trial, also found, the combination of glucosamine chondroitin-sulfate (GC) and methylsulfonylmethane (MSM) demonstrated a clinical benefit for patients with knee OA, compared with just the GC or placebo groups.[371] MSM supplementation appears to benefit skin health by reducing fine lines and wrinkles, and may improve hair and nail quality too. Additionally, emerging research suggests that MSM may one day help in the treatment of some types of cancer.[372]

Mushrooms Moulds & Yeasts

A mushroom is the fruiting body of a fungus. The kingdom of fungi also contains microorganisms called yeasts and moulds, and interestingly these are all genetically more closely related to animals than to plants.[373] [374]There are well over ten thousand varieties of mushrooms, but not all are edible. However, those that are edible and often used in supplements, include reishi, chaga, cordyceps, maitake, shiitake, maitake, and lion`s mane. When exposed to sunlight mushrooms are a great source of ergosterol, a provitamin form of vitamin D2, which is essential for calcium and phosphate absorption; this keeps bones, teeth, and muscles healthy. This unique characteristic of mushrooms, containing this particular form of vitamin D (D2), is only found in fungi and many plants that are actually contaminated with fungi or yeasts, themselves.[375] Mushrooms and fungi have a long and rich medicinal history, having been used in traditional remedies for centuries. Certain cultures even consume mushrooms for their hallucinogenic properties, often used in ancient religious rites for this reason alone. Moulds have contributed hugely to human health, particularly in recent times, and since one of the most important, momentous, but fortuitous of discoveries, that of penicillin by Alexander Fleming in 1928. Penicillins are a powerful group of antibiotics, first acquired from the common Penicillium moulds widely found in the environment. However, over time many bacteria have developed resistance to these penicillins, used to treat bacterial infections. In fact, the very first sign of evolved resistance was as long ago as 1940, when one strain of E coli, a commonplace bacterium found in the gut, began to produce an enzyme capable of inactivating the then recently discovered penicillin.[376] Before this discovery and the introduction of penicillin as an antimicrobial, there were no effective treatments for infections, and we were all reliant upon traditional remedies alone. Many suffered and often died from diseases such as pneumonia, gonorrhoea, rheumatic fever, and septicaemia. As a result of resistance, scientists are constantly on the lookout for novel antibacterial candidates. Many antibiotics are, in fact, produced by bacteria and fungi themselves, and these all have the capacity to kill or inhibit competing microbes.[377] Yeasts are also vital for our health, and play an important role in our microbiome, by keeping our digestive system in balance, assisting the absorption of essential vitamins and minerals from our foods, and helping our immune systems remain strong to fight disease.

N

Nettles- Urtica disoca

Also known as the common nettle or `stinger`, this perennial flowering plant has the characteristic, when raw, of causing contact dermatitis – skin irritation – by injecting two compounds, histamine and formic acid, into any unwitting subject that comes into contact with the tiny hairs found on the underside of the leaves — probably to protect the plant itself. This causes an unpleasant stinging sensation. However, if soaked or cooked properly, the humble nettle reveals its other attributes, including nutritional value, and a delicious irony spinach-like flavour with cucumber undertones; some have described the flavour as grassy, asparagus-woody, fishy, fermented, mint, and even citrus.[378] Nettles contain valuable nutrients, housing vitamins A and C, essential minerals, including iron, potassium, manganese, and calcium. The nettle has been used in traditional medicines by various cultures and is one of the most commonly used medicinal plants across the whole world. In Austria, for example, it is often consumed as a tea, to help ailments associated with inflammatory processes.[379] It was used in ancient Greece to treat coughs and arthritis, and some think Caesar's troops may have introduced the Roman nettle (U. pilulifera) into Britain, to deliberately sting themselves, maybe to keep warm, or as many think now, to relieve rheumatic pains![380] Its other benefits are thought to be wide-ranging, relating to both its antioxidant and antimicrobial properties.[381] Other benefits include uses as a diuretic, for the treatment of painful muscles and joints, and even eczema, gout, and anaemia. It has also been found to exert a healing effect on second degree burns.[382] Some German in-vitro studies have considered the possible immune-modulating effects of nettle leaf extracts on rheumatic diseases — so maybe the Romans were onto something.[383]

Noni- Morinda citrifolia

This small evergreen tree grows all the way from Australia across to South-eastern Asia. It is also abundant in Polynesia. Noni likes the mineral micronutrients from volcanic lava flows, which include, iron, magnesium, calcium, sodium, potassium, and phosphorus. These minerals help the tree grow and flourish. There are altogether 12 volcanoes in French Polynesia alone, and two of these are still active — Moua Pihaa and Rocard. Teahitia erupted in 1985 and Macdonald last erupted in 1989; so, plenty of landscape or habitat exists in those localities for this shrub to thrive and prosper. Historically, ethnomedical uses, included external applications and internal consumption for a variety of health issues alone, or sometimes in combinations with other herbs. Today it is the ripe fruit used in supplement form that is thought helpful for various chronic illnesses, including cancer treatment. In-vitro research findings have shown noni to have antioxidant, immune-stimulating, and tumour-killing properties, which may well warrant further study. However, human studies, thus far, have not shown noni has beneficial effects on any chronic health conditions. It is also unclear whether noni use may be associated with liver problems — particularly when used in medicinal quantities.[384] The fruit is a multiple fruit or collective fruit formed from clusters of flowers that coalesce into a single fruiting entity. The noni fruit has a pungent cheese-like aroma or even *vomit* tone, not very pleasant, nevertheless the fruit pulp powder does contain relevant quantities of vitamin C, niacin, iron, and potassium.[385]

O

Olive- Olea europaea

The Olive is a well-known, quintessential, native Mediterranean tree, widely grown for its edible fruits or drupes as they are known, and highly valued for its pressed oils, which are often used in cooking. However, for thousands of years olives were grown primarily for lamp oil, and the true origin of the plant is not really known. It is postulated by some, to hail from Syria or maybe sub-Saharan Africa.[386] Fossil records show the leaves of the olive tree dating back to the Palaeolithic and Neolithic periods, and there is even earlier evidence of cultivation, up to 8,000 years ago, in western Greece.[387] Olives are considered rich sources of vitamin E, containing large amounts of sodium, are rich in oleic acid (an omega-9 fatty acid), and polyphenols.[388] The black olive, in particular, contains anthocyanins, which might have beneficial health effects through their antioxidant properties.[389] Olive contains the polyphenol, known as oleuropein that is responsible for the bitter flavour. This compound is considered a powerful antioxidant, exhibiting anti-inflammatory and blood pressure-lowering effects.[390] Whilst more research is necessary, intake of olive leaf extracts may be related, in-vivo, to prevention of oxidative stress with several other associated health benefits.[391]

Omega-3 fatty acids

This group of polyunsaturated fatty acids (PUFAs) includes three important types, ALA -α-linolenic acid-, EPA -eicosapentaenoic acid-, and DHA -docosahexaenoic acid-; the latter two are the main types of polyunsaturated fats found in oily fish, which can help to lower the level of LDL cholesterol, often considered the bad type of cholesterol. ALA is the only essential fatty acid in this group, mainly found in plant foods, such as soybean, chia seeds, and avocados. The adequate intakes were covered in the ALA (Alpha-Linolenic Acid) description earlier in the book. EPA and DHA are not considered essential, as they can be synthesised from ALA, albeit inefficiently in the case of DHA. It is therefore beneficial to increase consumption of DHA in the diet, or through supplementation.[392] A 2018 study concluded that very few American children and older adults met even the lowest EPA and DHA intake requirements, despite being able to consume more balanced omega-6 to omega-3 ratios.[393] According to the European Food Safety Authority (EFSA), insufficient available data means a tolerable upper safety limit cannot be established for DHA, EPA, or DPA (an intermediary compound between DHA and EPA), either individually or in combination.[394]

Omega-6 fatty acids

This is the other type of polyunsaturated fat (PUFA), which has similar health benefits to the omega-3 fatty acids — these are found in most vegetable oils. Some types of omega-3 and omega-6 fats cannot be made in the body, therefore small amounts are considered essential in the diet. In 2009, The European Safety Authority (EFSA) published recommendations of 2 g per day of ALA and 250 mg per day of the long chain acids, EPA and DHA. The recommendation for omega-6 or linoleic acid (LA), an essential fatty acid, was 10 g per day. In 2002, the Food and Nutrition Board of the US Institute of Medicine established the following adequate intakes (AIs).[395]

Daily Adequate Intakes (AIs)

- 0-6 months: 4.4 g as total omega-6s present in human milk.
- 7-12 months: 4.6 g as total omega-6s present in human milk.
- 1-3 years: 7 g
- 4-8 years: 10 g
- 9-13 years: male 12 g: female 10 g
- 14-18 years: male 16 g: female 11 g
- 19-50 years: male 17 g
- 19-50 years: female 12 g
- Greater than 51 years: male 14 g: female 11 g
- Pregnant teens and women 13 g
- Breastfeeding teens and women 13 g

Omega-9 fatty acid

These unsaturated fatty acids, which include oleic and erucic acids, are not classed as essential in the diet, as both are such common components of animal fats and vegetable oils. Erucic acid is found in wallflower seeds, part of the cabbage family, rapeseed, and mustard seed oils. Oleic acid is the most common of all the fatty acids, a monounsaturated fat (MUFA), found in the highest levels in an olive oil rich, Mediterranean diet. Oleic acid is associated, when substituted in the diet for saturated fats, with a reduction in the risk of coronary heart disease; probably through modifying the cholesterol balance and lipid profiles.[396]

Oregano- Origanum vulgare

Oregano is an aromatic herb related to mint and marjoram, which is frequently employed in Mediterranean cooking, and was originally grown in Greece; it has many varieties, all with differing intensities and maybe properties too. As with many herbs, the traditional medicinal uses were deemed to be quite wide. In the Middle Ages it was valued to support wound healing and for relieving headaches, but these benefits are not corroborated currently by any good quality studies. However, there is some evidence oregano contains compounds that may help to reduce coughs and spasms, and oregano might also have antimicrobial properties — helping to fight bacteria, some viruses, fungi, intestinal worms, and other parasites. It might also help increase bile flow and improve digestion.[397] The essential oils responsible for some of these health properties, include carvacrol and thymol (thymol is also found in the herb thyme, discussed later in the book, as it is used in some proprietary preparations), and to a lesser extent the compounds, cymene and terpinene.[398] A 2016 study of oregano extracts showed possible tumour-suppressive properties, both in-vitro and in-vivo, and for the first time, in a breast cancer model.[399] Care should be taken if pregnant or breastfeeding, as extracts ingested in oral form and in medicinal quantities might be unsafe.[400]

P

Parsley-Petroselinum crispum

Parsley is a flowering plant originally from the central and eastern Mediterranean region — a familiar culinary herb. It contains vitamins A, B6 (or folate), and C. It is exceptionally rich in vitamin K, and is a rich source of iron, also containing some other important minerals.[401] In traditional and folk medicines, parsley has been used as a carminative (relieving flatulence), an antiseptic, anti-inflammatory, for the treatment of amenorrhea, dysmenorrhea (relating to menstrual problems), gastrointestinal disorders, and various dermatological diseases. The essential oils contain various active phenolics, including myristicin and apiol. These chemicals, along with the coumarin compounds it houses, have been shown to exhibit cytoprotective (protecting cells from damage), oestrogenic, diuretic, antibacterial, and antifungal properties.[402]

Pea- Pisum sativum

Peas are good sources of fibre, protein, vitamins A, B6, C, and K. Also, the essential minerals magnesium, phosphorus, copper, iron, and zinc, and the carotenoid, lutein. The yellow pea variety is especially protein-rich, often used in meat and dairy alternatives as a protein substitute.[403]

Pennyroyal- Mentha pulegium

Pennyroyal is another plant in the mint family, often smeared upon the body, by the ancient Greeks and Romans, to drive away fleas. These parasites are now known to have been carriers and transmitters — to humans — of typhus and the plague. Two thousand years ago the herb was used to terminate pregnancies, probably through causing liver damage in the mother; very unfortunately, death of the mother often followed.[404] In Medieval cultures it was used as a traditional remedy to relieve headaches, colicky pains, and to ease fevers, although to date there is no good evidence supporting these or any other claimed historical benefits.

Pepper- piper nigrum

Pepper is a flowering vine belonging to the large Piperaceae family of plants; it produces a dark red fruit with a single seed called a peppercorn, which darkens to a black colour when dried, and is often used as a spice in global cuisines. In food supplements, an alkaloid extract of pepper, known as piperine, is responsible for the pungency of pepper. This is used to increase the bioavailability of other compounds, notably curcumin, a polyphenol believed to have medicinal properties, which is obtained from the Indian flowering plant, Curcumina longa (turmeric). A research review of consumption, in humans, showed that piperine could hugely increase the bioavailability of curcumin by as much as a factor of around 20 times, or 2,000%, and could provide multiple enhanced health benefits as a result.[405] Historically 4,000 years ago, black pepper was also known as "black gold" — due to its trading value, and gold itself was frequently traded for pepper itself. In those days it was largely exported from the Indian west coast, now known as Kerala — where it was indigenously grown.[406]

Peppermint- Mentha piperitae

Peppermint is a popular cross between watermint and spearmint — used as a traditional remedy to relieve indigestion, tension headaches, and skin irritations. This herb grows throughout Europe and North America. Both the leaves and the essential oil from peppermint have been used in folk remedies, and nowadays the oils are frequently added to soap and cosmetic products for their pleasant fragrances. The scent is often described as cool, camphoraceous, sharp, often compared to the bouquet of menthol. Health benefits are mentioned in written records from ancient Greece, Rome, and Egypt, but it was not until the 1700s that peppermint was recognised as having distinctive qualities of its own. These days peppermint is used as a dietary supplement to treat irritable bowel syndrome (IBS), headaches, digestive problems, and even the common cold. The oil can also be used topically to relieve itching and muscle aches. Peppermint oil has been studied most extensively, though, for the relief of IBS, with one systematic review concluding that peppermint oil was an effective and safe treatment option in the short term.[407] So far, very few good quality studies have demonstrated that peppermint leaf is helpful for any other conditions.[408]

Pfaffia- Pfaffia paniculata

Pfaffia is also known as corango, suma, or Brazilian ginseng, but is not actually related to ginsengs at all, which are in the plant order Apiales. Pfaffias are in the order Caryophyllales, nevertheless they are believed to share some similar health-giving properties with ginseng. This large rambling ground vine provides traditional medicines, used in South America for generations to treat a wide range of ailments. The root contains self-protective compounds, known as phytochemicals, including soponins, glycosides, pfaffic acids, and other nortriterpene compounds — the acids were found to exert inhibitory effects on the growth of cultured tumour cells back in 1983.[409] The roots are also rich in nutrients, containing amino acids, trace minerals, such as iron, magnesium, and zinc, also vitamins A, B1, B2, B5, E, and K.[410] Pfaffia has been used traditionally to combat stress and fatigue, and to boost the immune system. Additionally, animal studies have shown promising intestinal anti-inflammatory properties.[411] Pfaffia powder is found in several food supplements.

Phosphorus-P

This element with atomic number 15 makes up nearly 1% of our body mass — it is mainly found in bones and teeth. Phosphorous fulfils a vital structural role, working synergistically with vitamin D to keep bones and teeth strong.[412] It is also vital for energy transportation and is used in every human cell, a component of the ATP molecule (adenosine triphosphate) that stores high levels of energy, and is synthesised by the mitochondria within our cells.[413] At various times of life we need differing amounts of phosphorus. The Recommended Dietary Allowances (RDAs) are 700 mg per day in adults. In children and teens aged 9 to 18, and women who are pregnant and breastfeeding, this increases to 1,250 mg per day. Young children and babies need lower and varying quantities based upon their ages.[414] The tolerable upper intake levels hover between about 3,000 mg and 4,000 mg per day, and from birth to 12 months of age, the only sources should be from breast milk, formula, and food. The Adequate Intakes for infants from birth to 12 months are equivalent to the average intake of phosphorus in healthy, breastfed infants. The full RDAs are shown below.[415]

Recommended Dietary Allowances (RDAs)

- 0-6 months: male 100 mg: female 100 mg
- 7-12 months: male 275 mg: female 275 mg
- 1-3 years: male 460 mg: female 460 mg
- 4-8 years: male 500 mg: female 500 mg
- 9-13 years: male 1,250 mg: female 1,250 mg
- 14-18 years: male 1,250 mg: female 1,250 mg; pregnancy 1,250 mg; lactation 1,250 mg
- 19 plus years: male 700 mg: female 700 mg; pregnancy 700 mg; lactation 700 mg

Pomegranate- Punica granatum

The pomegranate is a shrub that bears fruits, consisting of many seeds in little pockets of juice. The fruits themselves contain vitamins B6, C, and K, and some minerals. The seeds of the fruit are also a rich source of dietary fibre.[416] All parts of the shrub including the fruits, seeds, peel, roots, leaves, and flowers have been researched for their potential health benefits. The peel, itself, is rich in natural antioxidants, which are known to have positive effects on human health, as has been demonstrated by a great deal of ongoing research.[417] Pomegranates contain some of the highest levels of ellagic acid, one such natural phenolic antioxidant.[418] The pomegranate has been a symbol of fertility for thousands of years, but there are only a few animal studies that have demonstrated an increased or improved fertility so far; one using pomegranate peel.[419] Another, more recent animal study, in 2015, using pomegranate seed oil, concluded that positive or beneficial effects may be useful in assisted reproductive technology.[420] Historically, pomegranate has been used to treat many conditions, including wounds, sore throats, and heart conditions, and in Indian Ayurvedic medicine, the rind of the fruit and the bark of the pomegranate tree, itself, were used in traditional remedies to help with digestive functions. There is promising research on heart disease, showing that pomegranate antioxidants have unique effects on atherosclerotic plaques (arterial deposits), by improving high density lipoprotein activity — "the good or helpful cholesterol" — and pomegranate is beneficial in diabetic patients too, as the antioxidants lock onto pomegranate sugars.[421] A small 2011 clinical trial concluded that mouthwashes using extracts could be helpful in controlling dental plaque. A larger 2012 trial, with 100 dialysis patients, suggested that the juice might help to defend against infection, and found those patients given pomegranate juice three times a week for a whole year had fewer hospital visits for infections, and fewer signs of inflammation. It is worth noting that people with plant allergies may be allergic to pomegranate juice, and it still remains unclear whether pomegranate can interact unfavourably with some blood thinning medicines.[422]

Poppy- Papaver rhoeas

The poppy is a flowering, herbaceous plant, used by the ancient Egyptians to relieve pain. We now know the seeds contain traces of morphine and codeine; both are important prescription painkillers widely used today.[423] The petals were used as a folk remedy to ease asthma and soothe coughs. It is generally thought that the Sumerians, who hailed from modern day Iraq, cultivated poppies as far back as the end of the third millennium BC, and in those days their name for the plant extracts was "gil", translated as joy, and the poppy was known as "hul gil", the plant of joy.[424] The poppy has become an important symbol, reminding us of the sacrifices made by millions of soldiers and civilians during World War 1. A poem, "In Flanders Fields" was written by a Canadian doctor, Lieutenant Colonel John McCrae, to commemorate all the fallen during the Great War.[425]

Potassium-K

Potassium is a highly reactive metal element with atomic

number 19, which is an essential mineral constituting 0.2% of the human body mass. The positive ions are widely distributed in the body and are essential for a multitude of physiological processes, including muscle contractions, fluid balance regulation, nerve conduction, enzyme and other protein production. Potassium has been linked with blood pressure reduction, glucose and insulin regulation, and maintaining fluid balance.[426] It is found in all food types. Traditionally, we talk about bananas and tomatoes being high-potassium foods, which they are, but potassium is actually found in higher quantities per 100 g in the following: cocoa powder, wheat bran, soya, flounder and scallops, avocado, prunes, raisins and sultanas, sesame seeds, nuts (pistachios in particular), and parsley.[427] People with kidney problems need to take care with both potassium-rich foods and any extra supplementation, as they cannot remove, or excrete, excesses efficiently. Adequate Intakes vary according to age, climbing to 3,400 mg per day in adult men and 2,600 mg per day in adult women. Women who are pregnant or producing breast milk need slightly higher amounts, between 2,600 mg to 2,900 mg per day, and 2,500 mg to 2,800 mg per day, respectively. Those people who are low in potassium should only supplement based upon specific and individual needs, and under the guidance of a health professional.[428] High levels of potassium in the diet do not tend to pose a health risk under normal circumstances, as the kidneys have the capacity to eliminate any excess amounts through excretion in the urine. The Adequate Intakes for potassium are shown below.[429]

Adequate Intakes (AIs)

- 0-6 months: male 400 mg: female 400 mg
- 7-12 months: male 860 mg: female 860 mg
- 1-3 years: male 2,000 mg: female 2,000 mg
- 4-8 years: male 500 mg: female 500 mg
- 9-13 years: male 2,300 mg: female 2,300 mg
- 14-18 years: male 3,000 mg: female 2,300 mg; pregnancy

2,600 mg; lactation 2,500 mg
  - 19-50 years: male 3,400 mg: female 2,600 mg; pregnancy 2,900 mg; lactation 2,800 mg
  - 51 years plus: male 3,400 mg: female 2,600 mg

Prebiotics

Prebiotics were discussed under fructooligosaccharides; types of carbohydrate found in plants, which include chicory, onion, garlic, asparagus, banana, artichoke, leeks, barley, and dandelion greens. These may help to stimulate the growth of friendly bacteria in the gut.[430] The prebiotic discussion continued by talking about fibre, the part of our diets that is largely indigestible, but can ferment in the large bowel and provide nutrients for those beneficial bacteria and fungi to colonise the gut, thereby improving our microbiome.[431] The microbiome is vital for controlling digestion, and plays a vital, active role in the function of the immune system. The constituency of the microbiome is affected by internal stresses, but also outside factors, which include prebiotics and probiotics (please see the probiotics entry), antibiotics, and proton pump inhibitors (drugs that control stomach acidity). Imbalance in the gut microbiome may be related to the prevalence of irritable bowel disease and syndrome (IBD & IBS), and depression. The maternal microbiome can also affect immune responses, and consequently the development of the newborn child.[432] Expressed in a different manner; the gut microbiome is considered a major body organ that can be fed with prebiotics, thereby impacting our overall health in a beneficial way. Additionally, as there is such a great biome diversity in various populations, prebiotics appear to be a very convenient and cost-effective way to rebalance the human microbiome.[433]

Primrose- Primula vulgaris

The primrose is a flowering plant with at least 500 species, one of the earliest to flower in the spring; hence its name, which is derived from the Latin "Primus" meaning "First". It was originally native to Africa, Europe, and Asia, but is chiefly found in the Northern Hemisphere, preferring to grow in cooler climes. It is also known as the common primrose, but not to be confused with the evening primrose, which is a completely different plant. All parts of the primrose have been used for centuries for their painkilling and sedative benefits. Some people have also valued the primrose for presumed diuretic effects. The roots were particularly favoured in traditional herbal medicines. [434] Both the flowers and leaves are edible too.

Probiotics

Probiotics are a mixture of live organisms, intended to repopulate and improve the gut flora. Whilst prebiotic use might be more convenient in some ways, because of the ease of production and lower costs, probiotics and FMT (fecal microbiota transplantation) might provide therapeutic and diverse alterations for the intestinal microbiota, representing a potential treatment option for irritable bowel syndrome (IBS). [435] In 2011, one paper evaluated the evidence for probiotic efficacy, and concluded that preliminary evidence existed for most of the associated health claims. Subsequently, a 2012 meta-analysis concluded that probiotics were generally beneficial for the treatment and prevention of gastrointestinal diseases, but it was deemed important to take into account the specific species or strains used in the chosen treatment option.[436] A 2013 review corroborated these benefits, in general, concluding that there was sufficient supporting scientific evidence for the inclusion of probiotics in nutritional settings. The same review found certain health benefits, for which the best documented of those related to helping with bowel disorders, lactose intolerance, antibiotic-associated and infectious diarrhoea. Exposure to bacteria in early life may also provide a protective role against allergy, acting as a safe alternative stimulation for the developing infant immune system. [437] In 2017, an article in the Lancet added to the canon of information, expressing opinions that human research, so far, supported further study of these beneficial microbes for good mental health too.[438]

Proteases

Proteases are enzymes that help breakdown ingested proteins in the human intestines, so that their constituents, amino acids, can be used to make new proteins — both for human growth and the maintenance of all our cells and tissues.

Prune- dried plum- Prunus domestica

The prune is a dried plum, originally from wild stock of ancient origin. The plum has seeds (also known as stones, kernels, or pits), which are removed before drying for safe human consumption of the prune itself. The juice is rich in vitamin K, which keeps bones healthy and is vital for blood clotting and wound healing. The juice is also a moderate source of B vitamins and minerals, particularly potassium.[439] Prunes contain phytochemicals, numbers of phenolic acid compounds, and sorbitol. These along with the high fibre content, around 7%, may be responsible for the mild laxative effects prunes are famous for. These phenols also inhibit oxidation of "the bad cholesterol", called LDL, which may help to prevent progression of chronic diseases, such as heart disease and cancer. The high potassium content may also be beneficial for our cardiovascular health (excessive quantities, though, can cause heart muscle problems).[440] Those with kidney clearance problems should also be wary of immoderate amounts.

Psyllium- Plantago

This is a group of plants of the Plantago genus, which includes varieties colloquially known as blond plantain and psyllium, desert indianwheat, and ispaghul. The seeds and husks are used in traditional medicines and are now used as common dietary fibre (soluble) sources. There is some evidence showing oral consumption of blond psyllium is associated with improving stool consistency, thereby relieving constipation.[441]

Pumpkin seed- Cucurbita pepo

Pumpkin seeds are nutrient dense, containing omega-6 and omega-9 fatty acids, and are rich in vitamin B3 (niacin). Niacin deficiency causes the rare disease pellagra, ranging from a mild form, going virtually unnoticed, to a potentially fatal disease, which is fortunately now rare in the developed world. Pumpkin seeds also contain dietary fibre, and are rich in the minerals, manganese, magnesium, phosphorus, iron, and zinc.

Q

Quercetin

This is a compound with a bitter flavour belonging to the flavonoid group of polyphenols; it is mostly found in the roots and outer parts of fruits or vegetables (the skins). Some is also found in the leaves. Other polyphenols, include the astringent compounds known as tannins, which are used in numerous food applications, including beer clarification. Tannins are also useful as antidotes for metallic, alkaloidal, and glycosidic poisoning. The tannins act, as antidotes, by forming insoluble precipitates, thus avoiding the absorption of these dangerous toxins through the gut.[442] All polyphenols are important for plant functions — these are constantly under investigation for their possible benefits in humans, often because they have strong antioxidant effects.[443] Quercetin is an abundant flavonoid, found in many fruits, seeds and grains, capers, red onions, and kale. There are over 5,000 naturally occurring flavonoids. This particular compound, quercertin, is just one example frequently found in food supplements.

Quinoa- Chenopodium quinoa

Quinoa is a flowering plant belonging to the amaranth family, originally emanating from the Peruvian Andes, and grown for its nutritious seeds.[444] In the raw state, the seeds are rich sources of vitamins B1, B2, B6, and B9, but also contain several essential minerals, including manganese and phosphorus. However, we prefer to eat the seeds cooked, which subsequently causes some nutrient loss. Quinoa has become quite popular over the last decade or so, as it is a gluten-free and low in saturated fat alternative to rice — it has a higher protein content than rice too. Rice is a food staple for over 3 billion people worldwide.

R

Radish- Raphanus raphanis *subspecies* sativus

The radish is a herbaceous plant belonging to the mustard family (Brassicaceae), of which there are around 3,700 species. Whilst cultivation of radish started over 4,500 years ago in South-eastern Asia — radish also became popular in ancient Egypt, both as a salad plant and a source of oils (some varieties only). The root of this brassica is edible, with a peppery flavour, containing vitamins and minerals, particularly vitamin C. Vitamin C is important for immune system support, helping with wound healing, protection of cells, and maintaining skin, blood vessels, bones, and cartilage.[445]

Raspberry- Rubus idaeus

The raspberry is a hardy perennial, a member of the rose family, with around 200 different species. The raspberry is an aggregate fruit that has many drupelets, each considered a separate fruit. The European raspberry that many are familiar with is red, but there are American varieties which are black. The fruit contain high levels of vitamin C, small amounts of other vitamins, good fibre content, the mineral manganese, and some anthocyanin pigments (polyphenols). The polyphenols are under investigation for prospective health benefits, particularly for their potential role in reducing the risks associated with metabolically based chronic diseases.[446]

Red Clover- Trifolium pratense

Red clover belongs to the legume family. The flower tops are often used in traditional Indian medicines. They contain isoflavones, compounds similar in structure to oestrogen, which are found in dietary supplements, often taken to help with menopausal symptoms, high cholesterol levels, and osteoporosis. However, clear studies showing beneficial effects need to be conducted, as there is not enough current scientific evidence to determine the effectiveness of red clover compounds for any medical conditions.[447] Indeed, red clover may be contraindicated in some cases, particularly with respect to patients with oestrogen-dependent breast cancer (or at risk of), hormonal disorders, and during pregnancy or lactation.

Rosehip- Rosa rugosa

The wild fruit of the rosehip plant contains high levels of vitamin C and carotenoids. It is often used in food supplements.[448] A 2008 meta-analysis concluded that rosehip powder could have therapeutic value in reducing pain from osteoarthritis, but larger trials need to be conducted to both evaluate safety and establish efficacy.[449]

Rosemary- Salvia rosmarinus *or* Rosmarinus officinalis

Rosemary is a herb that has been traditionally used for treating epilepsy, poor circulation, and headaches. It was considered sacred by some ancient cultures. Wild rosemary was used in Arabic countries centuries ago for its perceived health benefits

— sometimes used for treating stomach infections, maybe due to its antimicrobial qualities. We now know ulcers are largely caused by bacterial invasion of the stomach lining by the Helicobacter Pylori bacterium, naturally this was not known in those days. Some studies have shown the polyphenols rosemary contains, carnosic acid and carnosol (essential oil constituents) possess antioxidant activity that may also be beneficial in prostate cancer control.[450]

Royal jelly

Royal jelly is also known as bee`s milk and comes from the salivary glands of worker honeybees. It is sold as a food supplement, but EFSA concluded in 2011, that health benefit claims, in humans, were unproven. It may also cause unwanted allergic reactions (many substances can of course) in those individuals who are vulnerable or susceptible. One review in 2012 concluded that there were benefits to royal jelly consumption, and these were probably attributable to the bioactive fatty acids, proteins, and other phenolic compounds bee`s milk contains.[451]

Rhubarb- Rheum rhabarbarum

The Latin binomial of rhubarb relates to the wild variety found in Siberia and China, which was initially harvested for its edible root. The precise culinary origin of the modern plant, belonging to the knotweed family, is not known, but we now enjoy the fleshy stalks, not the roots, for their nutrient value. We need to remember the leaves are to be avoided, as they contain high levels of oxalic acid, which is a toxic compound — also its salt, the compound calcium oxalate, is the most common component of kidney stones. Rhubarb contains high levels of vitamin K, several important minerals, and fibre.[452]

S

Sage- Salvia officinalis

This spice or herb, native to the Mediterranean, has a long history of medicinal use in Egyptian, Roman, and Greek cultures, often burned to promote healing. Like rosemary, sage contains the polyphenol antioxidant carnosic acid. It is now frequently taken as a dietary supplement for depression, memory loss, and digestive problems.[453] A 2017 review concluded that the cognitive-enhancing and protective effects of Salvia were promising and warranted further study.[454]

Selenium-Se

An element with atomic number 34, an essential micronutrient, part of two important amino acids in the human body (selenocysteine and selenomethionine).[455] The latter is found in Brazil nuts, cereal grains, and soybeans. Selenium is also found in mushrooms. It is essential for the thyroid gland and thyroxine-dependant cell function. Additionally, it is a vital cofactor for the chemical modification of some antioxidant enzymes, selenoproteins, which have elusive functions, possibly playing essential roles in numerous conditions and diseases.[456] Selenium intake has been falling in the UK for three decades now, even though we only need trace amounts. The UK Recommended Daily Allowance is currently 75 micrograms for men and 60 micrograms for women. The US recommended levels are slightly lower at 55 micrograms per day, unless pregnant or breastfeeding.[457] The full RDAs for selenium are shown below.

Recommended Dietary Allowances (RDAs)

- 0-6 months: male 15 mcg: female 15 mcg, Adequate Intake
- 7-12 months: male 20 mcg: female 20 mcg, Adequate Intake
- 1-3 years: male 20 mcg: female 20 mcg
- 4-8 years: male 30 mcg: female 30 mcg
- 9-13 years: male 40 mcg: female 40 mcg
- 14-18 years: male 55 mcg: female 55 mcg; pregnancy 60 mcg; lactation 70 mcg
- 19-50 years: male 55 mcg: female 55 mcg; pregnancy 60 mcg; lactation 70 mcg
- 51 years plus: male 55 mcg: female 55 mcg

Tolerable upper limits or upper intake levels for selenium vary according to age — these are shown below.

Upper limits (ULs)

- Birth-6 months: male 45 mcg: female 45 mcg
- 7-12 months: male 60 mcg: female 60 mcg
- 1-3 years: male 90 mcg: female 90 mcg
- 4-8 years: male 150 mcg: female 150 mcg
- 9-13 years: male 280 mcg: female 280 mcg
- 14-18 years: male 400 mcg: female 400 mcg; pregnant and lactating both 400 mcg
- 19 years plus: male 400 mcg: female 400 mcg; pregnant and lactating both 400 mcg

The only sources of selenium for infants should come from

breast milk, formula, and food.

Sodium-Na

This chemical element with atomic number 11 is essential for regulating blood volume and blood pressure. The main source is common salt (sodium chloride). Care needs to be taken not to consume too much, as this can have detrimental health repercussions. In fact, lowering salt intake is linked with a reduction in systolic blood pressure and hypertension.[458] NHS UK advises that adults should keep levels to no more than 2.4 grams of sodium per day (around a teaspoon [tsp.] or 6 grams of the actual compound, salt). The consumption necessary for children is age dependant and considered at lower levels in general. Babies need very little as their kidneys are underdeveloped and cannot process salt (sodium) properly.

Sorrel- Rumex acetosella or R acetosa

Sorrel is a perennial herb that likes to grow in grassland and at the edge of wood habitats. It is a member of the knotweed family. Another plant, Hibiscus sabdariffa, known as the "sorrel of the Caribbean", is a completely different plant originating from West Africa, found in the Caribbean as the main constituent of a very popular Christmas beverage. It is often flavoured with mint or ginger in West Africa, and sometimes referred to as "The national drink of Senegal". In Ghana it is known as "sobolo", and in Nigeria as "zobo". Rumex, itself, has been cultivated for centuries, containing vitamins A, C, and the mineral potassium. The flavour is described as having a sharp taste — this is due to its other components, compounds known as oxalates, which we have previously encountered.[459] Salts of oxalic acid (phytochemicals protecting the plants themselves) are also found in brassicas, parsley, and rhubarb. Too much oxalate in the human diet, as discussed previously under the rhubarb entry, can predispose to kidney stones; these are mainly composed of the compound calcium oxalate. The stone-forming reactions are enhanced when too little liquid is present as urine is processed by the kidneys.[460]

Soya bean- Glycine max

This legume is grown in vast quantities across the world to satisfy enormous human consumption. There is huge demand for a wide variety of soya-based products, including soy sauce, soy milk, tofu, soy flour, and oil. It is a great vegan alternative to milk, for those who are lactose intolerant or have dairy allergies. Other soya derived foods are Miso, a fermented paste used in Asian cooking, and Tempeh, an Indonesian cake made from the cooked beans. Soya provides many essential nutrients and has high levels of iron, manganese, and phosphorus, vitamin K, and several B vitamins, calcium, copper, magnesium, potassium, and zinc. It contains omega-6 (fatty acid), is protein rich, and contains fibre. It truly is a superfood, with the US growing the largest quantities until they were overtaken by Brazil in May 2020. Soya has historically been highly valued across the whole world, with archaeological records showing its cultivation several thousand years ago in Japan, China, and Korea.[461] Soya has been shown to lower total and bad LDL cholesterol levels,[462] and could be linked with reduced pre-menopausal breast cancer risks.[463] According to two 2016 systematic reviews and meta-analyses, soya may be associated with a reduced colorectal cancer risk,[464] and a small reduction in the risk of gastrointestinal cancer too.[465] Soybean oil can even provide environmentally friendly fuel for diesel engines, be turned into crayons, and has numerous other industrial applications.

Spinach- Spinacia oleracea

Spinach is a leafy plant, originally from Persia (now known as

Iran), and is traditionally favoured as a high iron content food, just ask "Popeye". Actually, spinach contains more manganese than iron, and is also exceptionally rich in vitamin K, which we have already seen is important for blood clotting /coagulation. In its raw form, spinach is also rich in vitamins A, B9, and C, and the mineral magnesium. It is considered a good source of vitamins B2, B6 and E, and the minerals, calcium, and potassium, as well as dietary fibre.[466] So, spinach truly is a nutritious plant with very high worldwide annual production. In 2018 alone, over 26 million tonnes were produced; China produces a whopping 24 million plus tonnes, and the US, coming in a distant second, but still in the silver medal position, producing over 323 thousand tonnes annually.[467]

Spirulina- Arthrospira platensis and maxima

This is a blue-green-algae used for centuries as a food in Mexico, and also several African countries. These days it is often used as a protein supplement and might be effective in reducing blood pressure in some people with high blood pressure.[468] It also contains the pseudovitamin B12, an inactive vitamin B12 analogue, with much smaller quantities of vitamin B12 itself. Several studies looking at current and potential clinical applications have shown positive effects in the treatment of allergic rhinitis, and possibly has cholesterol lowering effects too.[469]

Stevia- Stevia rebaudiana

Stevia is a plant belonging to the sunflower family, which is prized for its sweet-tasting leaves. It is also known as candyleaf for this reason. This perennial is native to Paraguay and the sweet-tasting chemicals are called steviol glycosides. Depending on the source, the leaves are thought to be around 100-200 times sweeter than sugar, containing *no calories* at all. Nowadays it is often used in food supplements — its safety having satisfied the US Food and Drug Administration in 2008, and subsequently the EU and EFSA in 2011. But for nearly 1,500 years, stevia leaves were valued as constituents found in traditional remedies for treating varied ailments, particularly by the indigenous Guarani people — natives of Paraguay and adjacent South American countries, including Bolivia, Argentina, and Brazil.[470]

St John`s Wort- Hypericum perforatum

St John`s wort is a flowering plant, celebrated as a traditional medicine for the treatment of mental health conditions and wounds for millennia — the name St. John's wort may refer to John the Baptist, the Christian preacher, born in the late 1st century BC. As of 2020, there has been little high-quality evidence to support treatment for depression. The US Food and Drug Administration (FDA) have not approved its usage either.[471] However, studies have yielded mixed results. A 2009 systematic review of 29 international studies suggested that St. John's wort could be better than a placebo (a substance that has no therapeutic effect, appearing identical to the study substance, and used as a control in testing new drugs), and at least as effective in treating major depression of a mild to moderate severity, when compared to standard prescription antidepressant drugs. Two other studies, in 2002 and 2011, did not demonstrate efficacy, though, when compared to placebo groups.[472] This herb is known to interact with several drugs, and consequently can cause serious side effects. The two compounds thought responsible for the pharmacological effects are hyperforin and hypercin, both plant phytochemicals (active self-protective compounds found in plants).[473]

Sulphur-S

Sulphur (Sulfur) is an essential element with atomic number 16. In prehistoric times, it is thought that sulphur was used by humans as one of the earliest tonic remedies to relieve digestive problems. Archaeological evidence has also uncovered numerous cave paintings using a reddish-brown pigment called cinnabar, which is a compound of mercury and sulphur (HgS).[474] As early as 2,000 years BC the ancient Egyptians burnt sulphur to bleach fabrics, and later the Greeks fumigated their homes with sulphur to eradicate pests.[475] It is also a key chemical, along with charcoal (carbon) and potassium nitrate, used to make gunpowder, discovered by the Chinese in around the 9th century AD. As a percentage of the human body, sulphur is the third most abundant mineral by weight, and according to the Jefferson National Linear Accelerator Laboratory, it is the 10th most abundant element in the whole universe. Six amino acids contain the essential element sulphur, which include methionine, cysteine, cystine, homocysteine, homocystine, and taurine;[476] with methionine and cysteine of particular importance in protein incorporation.[477] Sulphur, also, helps to maintain the shape of these amino acids with the proteins integrating them translating into cell rigidity in hair, nails, and skin. Sulphur is also a component of biotin — or vitamin H, vitamin B7, or vitamin B8, as it is sometimes known — insulin, and vitamin B1. Dietary sources are wide-ranging, and include eggs, dairy products, meat and poultry, fish, garlic, cabbage, nuts, onions, beans and split-peas, raspberries, and wheat germ. There is no Recommended Dietary Allowance (RDA) for sulphur, but there is a theoretical RDA for the essential amino acid that contains sulphur, which cannot be manufactured in the body without it, the essential amino acid methionine. This amino acid, together with other compounds, is also required to maintain the nitrogen balance in the human body. However, it is difficult to evaluate an actual RDA for methionine, as there is a requirement to assess both the nitrogen and sulphur balance together, and this has never been done in either humans or animals so far.[478]

T

Tansy- Tanacetum vulgare

Tansy is a flowering perennial belonging to the aster family, native to temperate European countries, except some of the Mediterranean islands and Siberia. It was subsequently introduced to many other parts of the world, sometimes referred to colloquially as golden buttons, cow bitter, and bitter buttons. It has a long history of use in traditional and folk medicines going back to the ancient Greeks. Tansy has been used variously to treat intestinal worms, digestive disorders, fevers, and sores. In the Middle-Ages and in high doses it was used to induce abortion and ironically in low doses to prevent miscarriages.[479] The plant contains toxins in the form of alkaloids and oils, which can cause contact dermatitis, and may be absorbed through the skin. In the past when tansy was used to lighten and purify the skin, we now know that this might have been ill-advised, as its toxic effects are considered cumulative, and long-term consumption can even cause death.[480] Thujone is the main toxic compound, a bitter tasting ketone, also consumed in the drink known as Absinthe — in years gone-by. This flavoured spirit contained various botanicals made from different herbs, which included grand wormwood (Artemesia absinthum), the main toxic culprit in this popular, highly alcoholic drink. It was originally distilled at the end of 18th century in Switzerland, and drunk widely until all countries had banned consumption by 1915.

However, common tansy has some natural benefits, with most of its compounds repelling the Colorado potato beetle (except for α-pinene, which to the contrary, actually attracts these beetles) — a major pest that has frequently devastated potato crops in Mexico and most states of the US over the years.[481] Research has shown beetle populations could be reduced by between 60 and 100 per cent, as the insects are thought to avoid many of the aromatic chemicals found in tansy oils.[482]

Tarragon- Artemisia dracunculus

Tarragon is a perennial herb belonging to the sunflower family, whose name means – little dragon – in French. This is a traditional Northern European aromatic herb used in a culinary setting since at least 500 BC. As a folk medicine it was used to treat toothache, digestive disorders, and many other maladies. It contains some nutrients, antioxidants, and the active ingredient estragole. However, very few modern studies have been conducted to verify any health claims in humans.

Tea Tree Oil- Melaleuca alternifolia

The leaves of the tea tree, also known as the Australian tea tree, and related to the myrtle, are sources of oil, used by the aboriginal people of Australia for thousands of years to treat cuts and wounds. The first recorded use of tea tree leaves for any medicinal purpose was documented by Lieutenant James Cook in 1770. The oil was used to treat scurvy amongst his sailors. This could not have worked though, as we have since discovered that vitamin C is required to treat scurvy, and all of his sailors were actually deficient in this essential vitamin — therefore tea tree oil usage was really a red herring. Later, Australian soldiers were issued with the oil — they used it as an antiseptic agent to treat wounds, initially in the 1930`s, and subsequently during World War II.[483] Today, tea tree oil is used externally, or topically, to treat acne, athlete`s foot, nail fungus, cuts, and insect bites, and to eliminate parasites, such as lice. Limited research does indicate that tea tree oil might well be helpful for acne, nail fungus, and athlete's foot. Topical application is rarely a problem, but oral ingestion is dangerous, and has been associated with confusion and loss of muscle coordination.[484]

Thyme- Thymus vulgaris

This herb is a member of the mint family, valued for its antimicrobial properties. It contains a range of compounds, which include thymol, an antiseptic used in many commercially produced mouthwashes, hand sanitisers, and acne medications. The ancient Greeks and Romans liked to burn bundles of thyme, both to summon courage, and cleanse their temples and homes. It was also used for embalming purposes by the Egyptians, and in the 1340s when the Black Death struck, millions of people turned to thyme for relief and protection, almost certainly to no avail — unfortunately. Thyme was included in many recipes before the days of refrigeration, as this may have afforded some protection from food spoiling and disease.[485] Thyme has also been used to kill parasitic worms and some fungal infections.[486]

Tomato- Solanum lycopersicum

Tomato plants produce fruits or berries, often red in colour, which contain compounds called lycopenes, and moderate amounts of vitamin C, other vitamins, minerals, and low levels of fat and protein. However, tomatoes have a generally low nutrient value, consisting of around 95% water. There is some evidence for the beneficial cardiovascular effects of lycopenes, and one 2018 review concluded that the compound was important in improving vascular function and involved in both the primary and secondary prevention of cardiovascular disorders.[487]

Turmeric-Curcuma longa

Turmeric is a herbaceous plant, a member of the ginger family, native to the Indian subcontinent and Southeast Asia. These regions provide the perfect growing conditions, in terms of rainfall and heat, for the roots to thrive and prosper. By virtue of its brilliant yellow colour, turmeric is also known as "Indian saffron" or the "golden spice" — its name, turmeric, is derived from the Latin word -terra merita-, meaning meritorious earth, for some esoteric reason. It is the roots that are used in cooking and are the source of curcumin, the active component often found in food supplements. When this is combined with another compound piperine, which is sourced from black pepper, there is a large increase in the bioavailability of curcumin itself — by up to 2,000 % within 45 minutes of oral ingestion.[488] Up to 4,000 years ago this flowering plant was grown and highly-regarded in culinary settings, also valued as a traditional medicine to purify blood. Today in Pakistan it is used as an anti-inflammatory, taken to help with gastrointestinal discomfort associated with irritable bowel syndrome (IBS), and to treat some other digestive disorders. It is sometimes applied to wounds in Afghanistan and Pakistan, for its perceived cleansing properties, also used in proprietary sunblock and face creams. It has always been employed as an important multipurpose remedy in traditional Chinese medicine and Indian Ayurveda, often referred to as the "Mother of All Healing."[489]

U

Uva ursi- Arctostaphylos uva-ursi

As suggested by the botanical name, this is a northern latitude loving woody shrub, known as the beargrape, as bears are quite partial to the fruit. The leaves and fruit were also considered important foods for the First Nation peoples of Canada, and the neighbouring Blackfoot Indians of the Blackfeet Tribe — from Montana.[490] It was used for centuries by the indigenous people of both Canada and south of the Arctic Circle as a traditional medicine to treat urinary tract inflammation, for constipation, and as a diuretic. Extracts have been shown to have some in-vitro antimicrobial effects too. Arbutin is the glycoside compound found in these extracts, considered the active chemical responsible for possible health benefits. Arbutin is also associated with beneficial antiviral in-vitro activity, acting against the herpes simplex virus type 2, the influenza virus A2, and the vaccinia virus (part of the poxvirus family).[491]

V

Valerian- Valeriana officinalis

This is a perennial flowering plant, native to Europe and Asia, but also found in North America. The roots and rhizomes have been used as medicines by the ancient Greeks and Romans. The famous Greek physician Hippocrates, who was considered the father of all medicine, was accustomed to prescribing valerian for his patients suffering with insomnia. Hippocrates described the aroma as pleasant, and valerian was widely used in perfumes of the time. Traditionally the herb was used medicinally as a diuretic, to aid digestion, to treat nervousness, trembling, headaches, and heart palpitations. The mild calming effects of valerian were even harnessed by the US government during World War 1 to treat shell shock or combat disorder as it is sometimes referred to — the root was also used as a sedative from 1820 to 1936, appearing in the US Pharmacopoeia, as an official remedy.[492] Today valerian is still used to help with insomnia, as a dietary supplement, and to treat anxiety, depression, and menopausal symptoms. There have been very few high-quality studies done in humans, and the evidence for helping with sleep problems is considered inconsistent at best. Additionally, there are very few good quality studies that demonstrate or can substantiate the efficacy of valerian for treating anxiety, depression, or menopausal symptoms. Studies do suggest, however, that most adults can ingest this herb safely, if used for short periods of time.[493]

Vanilla-Vanilla planifolia

Vanilla is a Mexican species of orchid. The pods contain the flavouring vanilla, which the Aztecs first developed a taste for back in the 1500s. Later in the 1700s, two visiting Spaniards Hernandez and Father Ignatius wrote about vanilla, but the claims they made with regards to medical benefits, which included aiding with digestion, treatment for head-colds, and catarrhs were exaggerated and unproven.[494] Modern studies show vanilla extracts contain antioxidants — these have potential applications for food preservation that could be employed in health food supplements, as nutraceuticals.[495]

Vervain- Verbena officinalis

Vervain is a semi-woody perennial flowering plant, sometimes known as the holy herb, as a widely circulated folklore story suggested that Jesus` wounds were treated with vervain after he was taken down from the cross. Vervain was used in ancient Roman times, when several species existed that still exist today, all with differing aromas and properties. The flowers, leaves, and essential oils have been used in traditional medicines for centuries to treat coughs and colds, shortness of breath associated with fevers, and a host of other conditions. Several compounds have been extracted from the plant, including verbenalin, hastatoside, caffeic acid, and various flavonoids; these may be responsible for some of the claimed medicinal benefits.[496]

W

Wintergreen- Gaultheria procumbens

Wintergreen belongs to a group of plants that we would call evergreens. These contain aromatic essential oils, sometimes described as strong and minty. The oils are chemically related to the active ingredient found in aspirin, in the form of methyl salicylate. Wintergreen is a herb that was frequently used in traditional or folk medicines to alleviate pain and ease fevers, but there are no good quality scientific studies that support all of the medicinal claims. It is currently used as a flavouring in some foods and pharmaceutical products.[497]

Woodruffe- Galium odaratum

Woodruffe is a perennial plant with small white flowers, which is native to many countries, but only sparsely naturalised in certain parts of the US and Canada.[498] Consumed as an infusion, this traditional herb has been used for centuries as a folk medicine to treat insomnia and digestive problems. Woodruff has also been taken for the treatment of insomnia and irritability, due to its tranquilizing effects. Again, when used as an infusion, it was believed to strengthen the stomach and remove obstructions from the colon. The main active compound responsible for its strong sweet-smelling aroma is coumarin — this is often used as a moth repellent, in potpourris, when the plant is dried. A potpourri is a combination of flowers, herbs, and spices, usually kept in a pot, jar or drawer, and used as a fragrance or repellent.

X

Xigua- Citrullus lanatus

Xigua is Chinese for watermelon, but these vine-like flowering plants were originally native to West Africa. The plants produce fruits that are approximately 90% water and contain a moderate amount of vitamin C, with traces of other vitamins and minerals. They also contain lycopene, a type of carotenoid, largely found in carrots, tomatoes, other vegetables, and red fruits.[499] More recently, global perspectives on carotenoids are recognising the roles these compounds may play in human health through influencing the biological roles of fatty acids, sugars, and proteins.[500]

Y

Yarrow- Achillea millefolium

Yarrow is a white flowering plant that grows in temperate regions, it is sometimes known as woundwort, old man's pepper, milfoil, and thousand-leaf. Traditionally, it has been used to treat a diverse range of conditions, including toothache and digestive problems. It has been used globally across widespread locations, including India, America, Canada, and Europe. In ancient Greece, Homer, the legendary Greek author, in his epic poem "The Iliad", refers to yarrow as a treatment to help with wound healing associated with the cuts and abrasions that many soldiers sustained on the battlefields of Troy. Yarrow contains chemicals with both antiseptic and painkilling properties. These include azulenes, isovaleric acid, and salicylic acid. Proazulene, itself, is a dark blue essential oil used to control the development of some types of mosquito larvae, and salicylic acid is the active ingredient in aspirin, an everyday painkiller, naturally sourced from willow trees. We spoke about plants and their self-protective properties in the introduction of this book, and have come across numerous examples, in many of the entries. The tactic that yarrow uses in supporting conservation and biological control is fascinating — it does not attempt to kill destructive insects directly, but instead releases chemicals, known as pheromones, to attract "good" predatory insects, that in turn prey upon the "pest" insects themselves. For this reason, yarrow is defined as a companion plant.[501]

Yerba maté - Ilex paraguariensis

Yerba is a species belonging to the holly (Ilex) genus, which is used to make a health drink called maté; an infusion using leaves and twigs, originally consumed by South American peoples. It contains high levels of flavonoids that are associated with a wealth of in-vitro studies showing antioxidant, anti-inflammatory, and cancer prevention properties, but sparse corroborating in-vivo research. Yerba maté beer and soft drinks have been chemically assayed, and have been found to contain three xanthines, including caffeine and theobromine (both known for their stimulant effects), and theophylline, which has certain bronchodilatory properties. Yerba also contains the essential minerals potassium, magnesium, and manganese.[502] Several studies have found yerba maté beverages and supplements could be helpful in the battle against obesity and might have cholesterol lowering benefits too.[503] The weight losses achieved by trial participants could be related to the flavonoid content of maté and its inhibitory effects in some fashion, and the cholesterol lowering properties may be related to its saponin content. A 2009 review of possible disease associations found a large variance in trial results, but still thought that hot, **not cold**, maté consumption could be linked with certain increased cancer risks.[504]

Yohimbe- Pausinystalia yohimbe

Yohimbe is an evergreen plant species native to western and central Africa, which has been used as a traditional medicine. It is often consumed, for its aphrodisiac properties, in the form of a tea made from the bark. Nowadays, it is found in various supplements to help with impotence, weight loss, chest pain, high blood pressure, and diabetic neuropathy. Yohimbe contains a compound called yohimbine, also known as quebrachine, which is a member of the alpha blocker class of drugs. Yohimbine chloride (a salt compound) is a US prescription drug used to help with erectile dysfunction.[505] Very few studies have been conducted to verify the efficacy of any supplements, but several have documented risks attached to consumption. Yohimbe has been linked with high blood pressure, anxiety, tachycardia (a condition that makes your heart beat more rapidly), heart attacks, and seizures, and can also cause stomach problems according to the California Poison Control System. This is based upon data gathered between 2000 and 2006.[506]

Z

Zinc-Zn

Zinc is an essential mineral with atomic number 30 that is involved in a host of vital human cellular metabolic processes. We need zinc in our diets. It is often added to foods and is frequently found in supplements. The bioavailability of zinc is better from animal products than from plant foods.[507] The European Food Standards Agency (EFSA) agrees with all of the following wording: zinc helps to support a healthy immune system, is needed for cell division, has antioxidative properties that help to scavenge free radicals, is required for the structure of healthy bones, is important for mental function and performance, is required for normal fertility, is needed for the development of the reproductive system, is required to maintain optimal muscle function, and helps to maintain a healthy male reproductive system. Zinc is an essential cofactor involved with fatty acid metabolism, impacting hormonal health, and promotes joint health and function. Men need zinc for a healthy prostate, and everyone needs zinc for a healthy thyroid. Zinc is also important for regulation of the acid-base balance. This element is found in high concentrations in the eye, as it is important for vision and dark adaptation. When we come in from the outdoors into a very dimly lit room, we find that we are hardly able to see our surroundings, initially, but as time goes by, we gradually adjust and can detect objects. This phenomenon is known as "dark adaptation," and generally takes about 20 to 30 minutes to reach its maximum, depending on the previous brightness and exposure of the individual to the outdoor surroundings.[508] Zinc is also necessary for the transport and metabolism of vitamin A in the body, and contributes to cell protection from the damage caused by free radicals (e.g., as a constituent of the enzyme superoxide dismutase). Zinc is a trace element vital for reactions involving around 100 enzymes relating to all the above processes and functions. It is found in a variety of foods, with oysters containing more per serving than any other source. Others are red meats and poultry, beans, whole grains, shellfish, nuts, cereals, and dairy products.

Phytates are acids found in whole-grain breads, cereals, legumes, nuts, and seeds — these are known to bind with zinc, thereby inhibiting its absorption. This process may be potentiated by calcium, which also reacts with phytates, by binding zinc to the resultant precipitate, consequently diminishing absorption further.[509] Phytates are the only substantial nutritional factors, sometimes referred to as antinutrient factors, which inhibit zinc absorption in this manner.[510] Advice for recommended daily consumption can vary from region to region, and below are the suggested Recommended Dietary Allowances (RDAs). The Adequate Intake (AI) for babies relates to the mean intake of healthy, breastfed infants.[511]

Recommended Dietary Allowances (RDAs)
- 0-6 months: male 2 mg: female 2 mg, Adequate Intake (AI)
- 7-12 months: male 3 mg: female 3 mg
- 1-3 years: male 3 mg: female 3 mg
- 4-8 years: male 5 mg: female 5 mg
- 9-13 years: male 8 mg: female 8 mg
- 14-18 years: male 11 mg: female 9 mg; pregnancy 12 mg; lactation 13 mg
- 19 plus years: male 11 mg: female 8 mg; pregnancy 11 mg; lactation 12 mg

Approximately 30-50% of those people who ingest too much alcohol are considered zinc deficient, as ethanol also decreases intestinal absorption.[512] The Tolerable Upper Intake Levels (ULs) are shown below for individuals who are not receiving specific treatments using zinc under the guidance of a health professional. High levels of zinc can also inhibit copper absorption, and reduce the absorption and action of penicillamine, a drug used to treat rheumatoid arthritis.[513]

Tolerable Upper Intake Levels for zinc (ULs)
- 0-6 months: male 4 mg: female 4 mg
- 7-12 months: male 5 mg: female 5 mg
- 1-3 years: male 7 mg: female 7 mg
- 4-8 years: male 12 mg: female 12 mg
- 9-13 years: male 23 mg: female 23 mg
- 14-18 years: male 34 mg: female 34 mg; pregnancy 34 mg; lactation 34 mg
- 19 plus years: male 40 mg: female 40 mg; pregnancy 40 mg; lactation 40 mg

CONCLUSION

Throughout this book we have tried to look at some important herbs and supplements, all the main vitamins and minerals, and have included their RDAs, AIs, and ULs where appropriate. Some of the most common herbs listed in the National Library of Medicine (NLM) herb garden are described with some appraisal of their traditional uses. There are around 75-100 herbs and flowers listed in the NLM though.[514] Apart from the traditional or folk treatments, modern medicine has discovered chemicals and compounds in these plants and herbs that can be isolated from them, and often have medicinal properties.[515] However, in recent times, some of the nutrients in foods have been reduced in concentration due to genetic engineering and poor soil quality. Sourcing or harvesting before natural ripening can also cause losses: this occurs mainly to enable global exportation without spoiling. All of these factors can impact overall chemical profiles. Additionally, intensive farming methods have altered soil biodiversity, leading to lowered vitamin and mineral content, particularly when compared to a few decades ago.[516]

Cooking

Cooking foods is helpful in many ways and some foods are not fit for human consumption unless cooked. The process of cooking involves high temperatures, which can kill most poisonous and detrimental bacteria sometimes found in foods like raw meat, poultry, fish, and eggs. The common bacteria that cause food-poisoning are campylobacter, salmonella, and listeria monocytogenes. Temperatures above circa 65°C (149°F), administered for the appropriate amount of time, kills most of these.

Cooking food improves digestion and can increase the absorption of many nutrients.[517] There is evidence that cooking was adopted more than 250,000 years ago, and over time has improved the net energy values available to us, from foods of both animal and plant origin.[518] For example, nettles are edible if soaked in cold water or cooked, which renders the stinging compounds ineffective — then nettles are good nutritious sources of vitamins A and C, as well as several minerals. One downside is that vitamin C is easily lost during cooking. In fact, vitamin C is lost through washing and cutting processes, as well as exposure to the air. Another example is egg protein, which is digested in the ilium (part of the small intestine) much more efficiently in cooked rather than raw form.[519] Many nutrients are reduced during cooking, including the water-soluble vitamins B and C, and the fat-soluble vitamin A. Fat-soluble vitamins D, E, and K are mostly unaffected by cooking. On average between 60% and 70% of essential minerals, sodium, potassium, phosphorus, calcium, magnesium, iron, zinc, manganese, and copper are also lost.[520] Cooking food does help us, though, to digest carbohydrate by initiating polysaccharide breakdown, which continues with the chewing process (our saliva contain amylase, the vital enzyme needed for this breakdown process). Cooking enhances the culinary experience — making food more appealing — by releasing flavours, improving food textures, and colours. However, another negative factor relating to nutrient loss is the valuable nutrients that are reduced or lost during the various preparation processes, before we even get to cooking food itself — through milling grains and peeling fruit and vegetables. Some accidental losses also occur during processing, storage, and transit. So, which of the nutrients briefly mentioned above are lost, and how exactly?[521]

Vitamin A

Vitamin A easily dissolves in fats and oils. As a result, when food is fried in oil, vitamin A leaches out from the food into the oil, only some of which we consume. Vitamin A is found in eggs, cod liver oil, orange and yellow fruits and vegetables, most dark green leafy vegetables, and many fortified products.

Vitamin B

Vitamin B is a water-soluble group of vitamins that is often discarded with water, so is lost before cooking processes to some extent.

Vitamin C

As already mentioned, vitamin C is easily destroyed during the cooking process. Cutting and peeling of vegetables and fruits causes some vitamin C loss, exacerbated by exposure to air for long periods, and the washing or rinsing of foods. Consequently, we need to think about the conservation of nutrients during preparation processes themselves.

Proteins

Proteins coagulate, denature, and soften, but if cooked for too long, water is lost — causing the food to become rubbery and difficult to digest.

Oils and fats

Cooking causes some separation of fats and fatty acids, thus diminishing their quality. Olive oil has a low smoking point and when used for cooking — particularly frying V can give off toxic fumes and impart bitter flavours to foods. Cooking fats for long periods causes oxidation and increases the production of harmful transfats (forms of unsaturated fats associated with several negative health effects), so is best avoided for these reasons alone.

Minerals

Most minerals, including zinc, iron, potassium, selenium, and others dissolve in water, or are carried in water, so become lost when food is cut, then washed and boiled. The used water is often discarded.

As we can see nutrients are lost in various manners from processing, storage, and transit, through to the preparation stages, with the discarding of the outer leaves and peelings, through to air exposure and the cooking processes themselves.

Alcohol

Too much alcohol consumption can cause nutritional deficiency in many ways.

Inhibition —

Alcohol decreases the secretion of some digestive enzymes from the pancreas.

Absorption —

Alcohol can damage the cells lining the stomach and intestines. This impairs the absorption of nutrients into the blood, also inhibiting fat absorption. The fat-soluble vitamins A, D, and E are particularly affected. Vitamins B (particularly B1, B12, and folic acid), C, and K are also found to be deficient in some alcoholics. Whilst many alcoholics are deficient in essential minerals, including zinc, which is important for normal hepatic metabolism,[522] deficiency is largely due to poor diets and other secondary alcohol-related problems.[523]

Structure —

Nutritional deficiency can alter the structure of cells. An example is folate deficiency and its relationship with altered small intestine cell formation. Ensuing cell damage can then cause further impairment with respect to absorption of water, glucose, sodium, and even folates themselves. High alcohol ingestion is associated with various malnutrition and medical complications, including liver damage, pancreatitis, brain dysfunction, and has potentially detrimental effects on foetal development, due to the toxicity of alcohol.

Neglect —

If we derive some or most of our calories from alcohol, a carbohydrate, we could deprive ourselves of the good nutrients available in other foods, which we will then not end up consuming. This is a form of calorific displacement.

Benefits —

Moderate drinking, however, may have beneficial effects on several other organs and systems. There may be decreased risks of some strokes, protection against diabetes type 2, a decrease in rheumatoid arthritis symptoms, improved cognition, decreased progression of liver disease (due to fibrosis in obese individuals), and improved renal function. Indeed, moderate alcohol consumption may be associated with an overall, small survival benefit, and has been shown to decrease some inflammatory biomarkers. This may well be the mechanism behind some of the protective effects.[524]

Absorption

We also need to be aware that some foods inhibit the absorption of others. For example, coffee can inhibit the absorption of iron, when consumed after a meal,[525] — zinc and copper have a relationship, where absorption of one inhibits the other, particularly when high levels are involved.[526] Phytates — naturally occurring compounds found in beans, grains and cereals, rice, and nuts — have a strong negative effect on zinc absorption from composite meals.[527]

All the information found in this book and accessed from various sources, I think, leads us inextricably to the conclusion that we need to retain balance in all the factors that affect us, obviously not just nutrition. But, as the German philosopher Ludwig Feuerbach posited, in 1848, in his famous phrase, "We are what we eat", nutrition is probably the most important, and is certainly the major driving force helping to keep body, mind, and soul healthy and together. I think it is largely agreed that we should not take Feuerbach completely literally, but the vision of connecting human essence, stress, and nutrition is vital, and further research into these areas could unlock even more links.[528] We are trying to put everything back together — we need to remember it was not apart in the first place.

Useful resources

UK based website for dietary recommendations

https://assets.publishing.service.gov.uk/government/uploads/system/uploads/attachment_data/file/618167/government_dietary_recommendations.pdf

US based website for nutrient recommendations

https://ods.od.nih.gov/HealthInformation/nutrientrecommendations.aspx

Canadian dietary guidelines

https://food-guide.canada.ca/en/guidelines/

Food and Agriculture Organization of the United Nations

https://www.fao.org/nutrition/education/food-dietary-guidelines/regions/europe/en/

European Food Safety Authority

https://www.efsa.europa.eu/en

---

[1] A. Vickers, C. Zollman and R. Lee, "Herbal medicine", *Western Journal of Medicine*, vol. 175, no. 2, pp. 125-128, 2001. Available: https://www.ncbi.nlm.nih.gov/pmc/articles/PMC1071505/. [Accessed: 24- Apr- 2020].

[2] "Compositae — The Plant List", *Theplantlist.org*, 2013. [Online]. Available: http://www.theplantlist.org/1.1/browse/A/Compositae/. [Accessed: 19- Jun- 2020].

[3] "Fabaceae | plant family", *Encyclopedia Britannica*. [Online]. Available: https://www.britannica.com/plant/Fabaceae. [Accessed: 19- Jun- 2020].

[4] H. Ardalani, A. Hadipanah and A. Sahebkar, "Medicinal Plants in the Treatment of Peptic Ulcer Disease: A Review", *Mini-Reviews in Medicinal Chemistry*, vol. 20, no. 8, pp. 662-702, 2020. Available: http://www.eurekaselect.com/177870/article. [Accessed: 4- May- 2020].

[5] "Vascular system | plant physiology", *Encyclopedia Britannica*, 2016. [Online]. Available: https://www.britannica.com/science/vascular-system. [Accessed: 21- May- 2020].

[6] R. Pallardy, "9 Plant Defense Mechanisms", *Encyclopedia Britannica*, 2020. [Online]. Available: https://www.britannica.com/list/botanical-barbarity-9-plant-defense-mechanisms. [Accessed: 25- Apr- 2020].

[7] H. Oz, "Nutrients, Infectious and Inflammatory Diseases". *Nutrients*, vol. 9, no. 10, p. 1085, 2017. Available: https://www.researchgate.net/publication/320176964_Nutrients_Infectious_and_Inflammatory_Diseases. [Accessed 28 May 2020].

[8] "Fact sheets - Malnutrition", *Who.int*, 2020. [Online]. Available: https://www.who.int/news-room/fact-sheets/detail/malnutrition. [Accessed: 02- Jan- 2022].

[9] "Global nutrition policy review 2016-2017: country progress in creating enabling policy environments for promoting healthy diets and nutrition", *Who.int*, 2018. [Online]. Available: https://www.who.int/publications-detail/9789241514873. [Accessed: 28- May- 2020].

[10] "FAO - News Article: Farming must change to feed the world", *Fao.org*, 2009. [Online]. Available: http://www.fao.org/news/story/en/item/9962/icode/. [Accessed: 28- May- 2020].

[11] "Food supplements", *Food Standards Agency*, 2018. [Online]. Available: https://www.food.gov.uk/business-guidance/food-supplements. [Accessed: 05- Apr- 2020].

[12] "General food law", *Food Standards Agency*, 2020. [Online]. Available: https://www.food.gov.uk/business-guidance/general-food-law. [Accessed: 05- Apr- 2020].

[13] V. Lobo, A. Patil, A. Phatak and N. Chandra, "Free Radicals, Antioxidants and Functional Foods: Impact on Human Health", *Phcogrev.com*, 2010. [Online]. Available: http://www.phcogrev.com/article/2010/4/8/1041030973-784770902. [Accessed: 14- May- 2020].

[14] M. Carlsen et al., "The total antioxidant content of more than 3100 foods, beverages, spices, herbs and supplements used worldwide", *Nutrition Journal*, vol. 9, no. 1, 2010. Available: https://www.ncbi.nlm.nih.gov/pmc/articles/PMC2841576/. [Accessed 28 June 2020].

[15] G. Drouin, J. Godin and B. Page, "The Genetics of Vitamin C Loss in Vertebrates", *Current Genomics*, vol. 12, no. 5, pp. 371-378, 2011. Available: https://www.ncbi.nlm.nih.gov/pmc/articles/PMC3145266/. [Accessed 14 April 2020].

[16] J. D'Mello, *Amino acids in higher plants*. Wallingford: CABI, 2015, pp. 88-93.

[17] H. Vickery and C. Schmidt, "The History of the Discovery of the Amino Acids.", *Chem-*

ical Reviews, vol. 9, no. 2, pp. 169-318, 1931. Available: https://pubs.acs.org/doi/pdf/10.1021/cr60033a001#. [Accessed 21 June 2020].

[18] "Cystine | amino acid", *Encyclopedia Britannica*, 2020. [Online]. Available: https://www.britannica.com/science/cystine. [Accessed: 21- Jun- 2020].

[19] "Arsenic, Boron, Nickel, Silicon, and Vanadium", *Ncbi.nlm.nih.gov*, 2001. [Online]. Available: https://www.ncbi.nlm.nih.gov/books/NBK222322/. [Accessed: 04- Apr- 2020].

[20] "Should You Take Dietary Supplements?", *NIH News in Health*, 2013. [Online]. Available: https://newsinhealth.nih.gov/2013/08/should-you-take-dietary-supplements. [Accessed: 29- Apr- 2020].

[21] "EFSA Panel on Dietetic Products, Nutrition and Allergies (NDA)", *Efsa.onlinelibrary.wiley.com*, 2009. [Online]. Available: https://efsa.onlinelibrary.wiley.com/doi/epdf/10.2903/j.efsa.2009.1226. [Accessed: 07- May- 2021].

[22] G. Brittenham, "Safety of Iron Fortification and Supplementation in Malaria-Endemic Areas", *Meeting Micronutrient Requirements for Health and Development*, pp. 117-127, 2012. Available: https://www.ncbi.nlm.nih.gov/pmc/articles/PMC4353606/. [Accessed 14 April 2020].

[23] *Govinfo.gov*, 2016. [Online]. Available: https://www.govinfo.gov/content/pkg/FR-2016-05-27/pdf/2016-11867.pdf. [Accessed: 29- Apr- 2020].

[24] "A Consumer's Guide to the DRIs (Dietary Reference Intakes) - Canada.ca", *Canada.ca*, 2020. [Online]. Available: https://www.canada.ca/en/health-canada/services/food-nutrition/healthy-eating/dietary-reference-intakes/consumer-guide-dris-dietary-reference-intakes.html. [Accessed: 29- Apr- 2020].

[25] *Efsa.europa.eu*, 2006. [Online]. Available: http://www.efsa.europa.eu/sites/default/files/efsa_rep/blobserver_assets/ndatolerableuil.pdf. [Accessed: 29- Apr- 2020].

[26] G. Wu, F. Bazer, T. Cudd, C. Meininger and T. Spencer, "Maternal Nutrition and Fetal Development", *The Journal of Nutrition*, vol. 134, no. 9, pp. 2169-2172, 2004. Available: https://academic.oup.com/jn/article/134/9/2169/4688801#112060753. [Accessed 27 June 2020].

[27] M. Kramer and R. Kakuma, "Energy and protein intake in pregnancy." *Cochrane Database Syst Rev*. 2003;(4):CD000032. https://pubmed.ncbi.nlm.nih.gov/14583907/. [Accessed: 10- May- 2020]

[28] F. Marangoni et al, "Maternal Diet and Nutrient Requirements in Pregnancy and Breastfeeding. An Italian Consensus Document", *Nutrients*, vol. 8, no. 10, p. 629, 2016. Available: https://www.ncbi.nlm.nih.gov/pmc/articles/PMC5084016/. [Accessed 10 May 2020].

[29] K. Crider, L. Bailey and R. Berry, "Folic Acid Food Fortification—Its History, Effect, Concerns, and Future Directions", *Nutrients*, vol. 3, no. 3, pp. 370-384, 2011. Available: https://www.ncbi.nlm.nih.gov/pmc/articles/PMC3257747/. [Accessed 10 May 2020].

[30] P. Haggarty, "UK introduces folic acid fortification of flour to prevent neural tube defects", The Lancet, vol. 398, no. 10307, pp. 1199-1201, 2021. Available: https://doi.org/10.1016/S0140-6736(21)02134-6. [Accessed 2 January 2022].

[31] L. Adair, "Long-Term Consequences of Nutrition and Growth in Early Childhood and Possible Preventive Interventions", *International Nutrition: Achieving Millennium Goals and Beyond*, pp. 111-120, 2014. Available: https://pubmed.ncbi.nlm.nih.gov/24504211/. [Accessed 10 May 2020].

[32] S. Bastos Maia et al., "Vitamin A and Pregnancy: A Narrative Review", *Nutrients*, vol. 11, no. 3, p. 681, 2019. Available: https://www.ncbi.nlm.nih.gov/pmc/articles/PMC6470929/. [Accessed 10 May 2020].

[33] S. Bilbo, G. Wray, S. Perkins and W. Parker, "Reconstitution of the human biome as the most reasonable solution for epidemics of allergic and autoimmune diseases", *Medical Hypotheses*, vol. 77, no. 4, pp. 494-504, 2011. Available: https://www.sciencedirect.com/science/article/abs/pii/S0306987711002775. Accessed 4 May 2020].

[34] P. Turnbaugh, R. Ley, M. Hamady, C. Fraser-Liggett, R. Knight and J. Gordon, "The Human Microbiome Project", *Nature*, vol. 449, no. 7164, pp. 804-810, 2007. Available: https://www.nature.com/articles/nature06244. [Accessed 25 June 2020].

[35] P. D'Adamo and C. Whitney, *EAT RIGHT 4 YOUR TYPE*. London: ARROW BOOKS, 2017, pp. 16,34,35,39,59,62 and 63.

[36] J. Zhao et al., "Relationship between the ABO Blood Group and the COVID-19 Susceptibility", 2020. Available: https://www.medrxiv.org/content/10.1101/2020.03.11.20031096v2. [Accessed 25 June 2020].

[37] Christian Yates, U. and Shaw, N., 2021. All world's coronavirus could fit into a Coke can - with room to spare. [online] HullLive. Available at: <https://www.bristolpost.co.uk/news/uk-world-news/worlds-coronavirus-could-fit-coke-4986895> [Accessed 19 February 2021].

[38] P. D`Adamo, "The Blood Type Diets : Blood Type and Your Health", *Dadamo.com*, 2019. [Online]. Available: https://dadamo.com/txt/index.pl?1001. [Accessed: 28- Jun- 2020].

[39] *Efsa.europa.eu*, 2010. [Online]. Available: https://www.efsa.europa.eu/sites/default/files/consultation/consultation/nda100928.pdf. [Accessed: 29- Apr- 2020].

[40] S. Becattini, Y. Taur and E. Pamer, "Antibiotic-Induced Changes in the Intestinal Microbiota and Disease", *Trends in Molecular Medicine*, vol. 22, no. 6, pp. 458-478, 2016. Available: https://doi.org/10.1016/j.molmed.2016.04.003. [Accessed 29 May 2020].

[41] D. Stekel, "First report of antimicrobial resistance pre-dates penicillin", *Nature*, vol. 562, no. 7726, pp. 192-192, 2018. Available: https://www.nature.com/articles/d41586-018-06983-0. [Accessed 29 May 2020].

[42] E. ABRAHAM and E. CHAIN, "An Enzyme from Bacteria able to Destroy Penicillin", *Nature*, vol. 146, no. 3713, pp. 837-837, 1940. Available: https://pubmed.ncbi.nlm.nih.gov/3055168/. [Accessed 29 May 2020].

[43] K. Honda and D. Littman, "The microbiota in adaptive immune homeostasis and disease." *Nature* **535**, 75–84 (2016). [Online]. Available: https://doi.org/10.1038/nature18848 [Accessed: 13- April- 2020].

[44] "The Perrin Technique: South Manchester & Cheshire", *The Village Osteopaths*. [Online]. Available: https://www.thevillageosteopaths.co.uk/the-perrin-technique. [Accessed: 28- Jun- 2020].

[45] S. Abeles and D. Pride, "Molecular Bases and Role of Viruses in the Human Microbiome", *sciencedirect.com*, 2014. [Online]. Available: https://doi.org/10.1016/j.jmb.2014.07.002. [Accessed: 27- May- 2020].

[46] C. Zimmer, "Ancient Viruses Are Buried in Your DNA", *Nytimes.com*, 2017. [Online]. Available: https://www.nytimes.com/2017/10/04/science/ancient-viruses-dna-genome.html. [Accessed: 27- May- 2020]

[47] "Human Genome Project FAQ", *Genome.gov*, 2020. [Online]. Available: https://www.genome.gov/human-genome-project/Completion-FAQ. [Accessed: 28- May- 2020].

[48] Aiewsakun and A. Katzourakis, "Marine origin of retroviruses in the early Palaeozoic Era", *Nature Communications*, vol. 8, no. 1, 2017. Available: https://pubmed.ncbi.nlm.nih.gov/28071651/. [Accessed 28 May 2020].

[49] "Healthy body", *nhs.uk*, 2020. [Online]. Available: https://www.nhs.uk/live-well/healthy-body/. [Accessed: 05- Apr- 2020].

[50] [Online]. Available: https://www.nhs.uk/change4life/food-facts/sugar. [Accessed: 21- Jun- 2020].

[51] S. Boseley, "'Ultra-processed' products now half of all UK family food purchases", *the Guardian*, 2018. [Online]. Available: https://www.theguardian.com/science/2018/feb/02/ultra-processed-products-now-half-of-all-uk-family-food-purchases. [Accessed: 21- Jun- 2020].

[52] Z. Zhao and A. Ross, "Retinoic Acid Repletion Restores the Number of Leukocytes and Their Subsets and Stimulates Natural Cytotoxicity in Vitamin A-Deficient Rats", *The Journal of Nutrition*, vol. 125, no. 8, pp. 2064-2073, 1995. Available: https://pubmed.ncbi.nlm.nih.gov/7643240/. [Accessed 28 May 2020].

[53] M. Zhong, R. Kawaguchi, M. Kassai and H. Sun, "Retina, Retinol, Retinal and the Natural History of Vitamin A as a Light Sensor", *Nutrients*, vol. 4, no. 12, pp. 2069-2096, 2012. Available: https://www.mdpi.com/2072-6643/4/12/2069. [Accessed 28 May 2020].

[54] R. Semba, "On the 'Discovery' of Vitamin A", *Annals of Nutrition and Metabolism*, vol. 61, no. 3, pp. 192-198, 2012. Available: https://www.karger.com/Article/Abstract/343124. [Accessed 28 May 2020].

[55] "Lunin, Nikolai Ivanovich", *Clever-geek.github.io*, 2020. [Online]. Available: https://clever-geek.github.io/articles/350424/index.html. [Accessed: 28- May- 2020].

[56] *Apps.who.int*, 2020. [Online]. Available: https://apps.who.int/iris/bitstream/handle/10665/44110/9789241598019_eng.pdf?ua=1. [Accessed: 10- Apr- 2020].

[57] "Vitamin A", *Ncbi.nlm.nih.gov*, 2001. [Online]. Available: https://www.ncbi.nlm.nih.gov/books/NBK222318/ [Accessed: 30- Apr- 2021].

[58] A. Schauss et al., "Antioxidant Capacity and Other Bioactivities of the Freeze-Dried Ama-

zonian Palm Berry,Euterpe oleraceaeMart. (Acai)", *Journal of Agricultural and Food Chemistry*, vol. 54, no. 22, pp. 8604-8610, 2006. Available: https://pubs.acs.org/doi/10.1021/jf0609779. [Accessed 8 April 2020].

[59] *Nccih.nih.gov*, 2016. [Online]. Available: https://www.nccih.nih.gov/health/acai. [Accessed: 21- May- 2020].

[60] A. Prakash and R. Baskaran, "Acerola, an untapped functional superfruit: a review on latest frontiers", *Journal of Food Science and Technology*, vol. 55, no. 9, pp. 3373-3384, 2018. Available: https://www.ncbi.nlm.nih.gov/pmc/articles/PMC6098779/. [Accessed 8 April 2020].

[61] T. Mezadri, D. Villaño, M. Fernández-Pachón, M. García-Parrilla and A. Troncoso, "Antioxidant compounds and antioxidant activity in acerola (Malpighia emarginata DC.) fruits and derivatives", *Journal of Food Composition and Analysis*, vol. 21, no. 4, pp. 282-290, 2008. Available: https://www.sciencedirect.com/science/article/abs/pii/S0889157508000227/. [Accessed 13 April 2020].

[62] "Office of Dietary Supplements - Manganese", *Ods.od.nih.gov*, 2020. [Online]. Available: https://ods.od.nih.gov/factsheets/Manganese-HealthProfessional/. [Accessed: 08- Apr- 2020].

[63] J. Mann, *How to poison your spouse the natural way*. [Christchurch, N.Z.]: JDM & Associates, 2004, p. 45.

[64] "Alfalfa: MedlinePlus Supplements", *Medlineplus.gov*, 2019. [Online]. Available: https://medlineplus.gov/druginfo/natural/19.html. [Accessed: 26- May- 2020].

[65] "Five Original Writing Systems", *Chemsites.chem.rutgers.edu*, 2020. [Online]. Available: http://chemsites.chem.rutgers.edu/~kyc/Five%20Original%20Writing%20Systems.html. [Accessed: 21- May- 2020].

[66] "The History of Aloe Vera", *Atalayabio.com*, 2020. [Online]. Available: https://www.atalayabio.com/en/the-history-of-aloe-vera. [Accessed: 21- May- 2020].

[67] A. Surjushe, R. Vasani and D. Saple, "Aloe vera: A short review", *Indian Journal of Dermatology*, vol. 53, no. 4, p. 163, 2008. Available: https://www.ncbi.nlm.nih.gov/pmc/articles/PMC2763764/. [Accessed 10 April 2020].

[68] *Nccih.nih.gov*, 2020. [Online]. Available: https://www.nccih.nih.gov/health/aloe-vera. [Accessed: 21- May- 2020].

[69] "Office of Dietary Supplements - Omega-3 Fatty Acids", *Ods.od.nih.gov*, 2019. [Online]. Available: https://ods.od.nih.gov/factsheets/Omega3FattyAcids-HealthProfessional/. [Accessed: 30- Apr- 2020].

[70] B. Salehi et al., "Insights on the Use of α-Lipoic Acid for Therapeutic Purposes", *Biomolecules*, vol. 9, no. 8, p. 356, 2019. Available: https://www.ncbi.nlm.nih.gov/pmc/articles/PMC6723188/. [Accessed 30 April 2020].

[71] C. Carol S. Johnston, "Vinegar: Medicinal Uses and Antiglycemic Effect", *PubMed Central (PMC)*, 2006. [Online]. Available: https://www.ncbi.nlm.nih.gov/pmc/articles/PMC1785201/. [Accessed: 30- Apr- 2020].

[72] C. Ulbricht, "Natural Standard Herb & Supplement Guide - 1st Edition" p. 59, *Elsevier.com*, 2010. [Online]. Available: https://www.elsevier.com/books/natural-standard-herb-and-supplement-guide/unknown/978-0-323-07295-3. [Accessed: 21- May- 2020].

[73] M. Cameron and S. Chrubasik, "Topical herbal therapies for treating osteoarthritis", *Cochrane Database of Systematic Reviews*, 2013. Available: https://pubmed.ncbi.nlm.nih.gov/23728701/. [Accessed 12 May 2020].

[74] "Arnica: MedlinePlus Supplements", *Medlineplus.gov, 2019*. Online]. Available: https://medlineplus.gov/druginfo/natural/721.html. [Accessed: 12- May- 2020].

[75] "Hildegard's History of Arnica - Healthy Hildegard", *Healthy Hildegard*, 2020. [Online]. Available: https://www.healthyhildegard.com/history-of-arnica/. [Accessed: 30- May- 2020].

[76] L. Stradley, "Artichokes History", *What's Cooking America*, 2020. [Online]. Available: https://whatscookingamerica.net/History/ArtichokeHistory.htm. [Accessed: 30- May- 2020].

[77] M. Elsebai, A. Mocan and A. Atanasov, "Cynaropicrin: A Comprehensive Research Review and Therapeutic Potential As an Anti-Hepatitis C Virus Agent", *Frontiers in Pharmacology*, vol. 7, 2016. Available: https://www.ncbi.nlm.nih.gov/pmc/articles/PMC5143615/. [Accessed 10 April 2020].

[78] N Singh, Narendra, M Bhalla, P de Jager, and M Gilca, (2011). "An Overview on Ashwagandha: A Rasayana (Rejuvenator) of Ayurveda." *African journal of traditional, complementary, and alternative medicines* : AJTCAM / African Networks on Ethnomedicines. 8. 208-13. 10.4314/ajtcam.v8i5S.9. [Accessed: 10- April- 2020]

[79] "Ashwagandha: MedlinePlus Supplements", *Medlineplus.gov, 2019*. [Online]. Available: https://medlineplus.gov/druginfo/natural/953.html. [Accessed: 26- Apr- 2020].

[80] *Nccih.nih.gov*, 2016. [Online]. Available: https://www.nccih.nih.gov/health/astragalus. [Accessed: 21- May- 2020].

[81] Y. Zheng, W. Ren, L. Zhang, Y. Zhang, D. Liu and Y. Liu, "A Review of the Pharmacological Action of Astragalus Polysaccharide", *Frontiers in Pharmacology*, vol. 11, 2020. Available: https://www.ncbi.nlm.nih.gov/pmc/articles/PMC7105737/. [Accessed 21 May 2020].

[82] "Safety of astaxanthin for its use as a novel food in food supplements", *European Food Safety Authority*, 2019. [Online]. Available: https://www.efsa.europa.eu/en/efsajournal/pub/5993. [Accessed: 10- Apr- 2020].

[83] P. Oelrichs, J. Ng, A. Seawright, A. Ward, L. Schäffeler and J. Macleod, "Isolation and identification of a compound from avocado (Persea americana) leaves which causes necrosis of the acinar epithelium of the lactating mammary gland and the myocardium", *Natural Toxins*, vol. 3, no. 5, pp. 344-349, 1995. Available: https://pubmed.ncbi.nlm.nih.gov/8581318/. [Accessed 30 May 2020].

[84] A. Chopra et al., "Ayurvedic medicine offers a good alternative to glucosamine and celecoxib in the treatment of symptomatic knee osteoarthritis: a randomized, double-blind, controlled equivalence drug trial", *Rheumatology*, vol. 52, no. 8, pp. 1408-1417, 2013. Avail-

able: https://academic.oup.com/rheumatology/article/52/8/1408/1790450. [Accessed 13 May 2020].

[85] D. Furst et al., "Double-Blind, Randomized, Controlled, Pilot Study Comparing Classic Ayurvedic Medicine, Methotrexate, and Their Combination in Rheumatoid Arthritis", *Journal of Clinical Rheumatology*, vol. 17, no. 1, pp. 185-192, 2011. Available: https://pubmed.ncbi.nlm.nih.gov/21617554/. [Accessed 13 May 2020].

[86] K. Sridharan, R. Mohan, S. Ramaratnam and D. Panneerselvam, "Ayurvedic treatments for diabetes mellitus", *Cochrane Database of Systematic Reviews*, 2011. Available: https://www.ncbi.nlm.nih.gov/pmc/articles/PMC3718571/. [Accessed 13 May 2020].

[87] M. Baliga, N. Joseph, M. Venkataranganna, A. Saxena, V. Ponemone and R. Fayad, "Curcumin, an active component of turmeric in the prevention and treatment of ulcerative colitis: preclinical and clinical observations", *Food & Function*, vol. 3, no. 11, p. 1109, 2012. Available: https://pubmed.ncbi.nlm.nih.gov/22833299/. [Accessed 13 May 2020].

[88] *Nccih.nih.gov*, 2019. [Online]. Available: https://www.nccih.nih.gov/health/ayurvedic-medicine-in-depth. [Accessed: 13- May- 2020].

[89] P. May, "Vitamin B1 (Thiamine)- Molecule of the Month - September 2017",*Chm.bris.ac.uk*, 2020. [Online]. Available: http://www.chm.bris.ac.uk/motm/vitaminB1/vitaminb1h.htm. [Accessed: 31- May- 2020].

[90] "Beriberi | Genetic and Rare Diseases Information Center (GARD) – an NCATS Program", *Rarediseases.info.nih.gov*, 2020. [Online]. Available: https://rarediseases.info.nih.gov/diseases/9948/beriberi. [Accessed: 11- Apr- 2020].

[91] "Benfotiamine, thiamine monophosphate chloride and thiamine pyrophosphate chloride, as sources of vitamin B1 added for nutritional purposes to food supplements - Scientific Opinion of the Panel on Food Additives and Nutrient Sources added to Food (ANS)", *EFSA Journal*, vol. 6, no. 11, p. 864, 2008. Available: https://efsa.onlinelibrary.wiley.com/doi/epdf/10.2903/j.efsa.2008.864. [Accessed 11 April 2020].

[92] "Office of Dietary Supplements - Thiamin", *Ods.od.nih.gov,* 2020. [Online]. Available: https://ods.od.nih.gov/factsheets/Thiamin-HealthProfessional/. [Accessed: 30- Apr- 2020].

[93] R. Sherwood, "Riboflavin Deficiency - an overview | ScienceDirect Topics", *Sciencedirect.com*, 2020. [Online]. Available: https://www.sciencedirect.com/topics/medicine-and-dentistry/riboflavin-deficiency. [Accessed: 31- May- 2020].

[94] "Vitamin B Complex - American Chemical Society National Historic Chemical Landmarks. The Vitamin B Complex.", *American Chemical Society*, 2016. [Online]. Available: https://www.acs.org/content/acs/en/education/whatischemistry/landmarks/vitamin-b-complex.html. [Accessed: 31- May- 2020].

[95] "Office of Dietary Supplements - Riboflavin", *Ods.od.nih.gov*, 2020. [Online]. Available: https://ods.od.nih.gov/factsheets/Riboflavin-HealthProfessional/#h5. [Accessed: 11- Apr- 2020].

[96] T. Meštrović, "Niacin History", *News-Medical.net*, 2018. [Online]. Available: https://www.news-medical.net/health/Niacin-History.aspx . [Accessed: 31- May- 2020].

[97] "Office of Dietary Supplements - Niacin", *Ods.od.nih.gov*, 2020. [Online]. Available: https://ods.od.nih.gov/factsheets/Niacin-HealthProfessional/. [Accessed: 30- Apr- 2020].

[98] "Scientific Opinion on the substantiation of health claims related to pantothenic acid", *Efsa.onlinelibrary.wiley.com*, 2010. [Online]. Available: https://efsa.onlinelibrary.wiley.com/doi/epdf/10.2903/j.efsa.2010.1758. [Accessed: 11- Apr- 2020].

[99] M. Davidson, "Molecular Expressions: The Vitamin Collection - Pantothenic Acid (Pantothenate, Vitamin B-5)", *Micro.magnet.fsu.edu*, 2018. [Online]. Available: https://micro.magnet.fsu.edu/vitamins/pages/pantothenate.html. [Accessed: 31- May- 2020].

[100] "Office of Dietary Supplements - Pantothenic Acid", *Ods.od.nih.gov*, 2020. [Online]. Available: https://ods.od.nih.gov/factsheets/PantothenicAcid-HealthProfessional/. [Accessed: 30- Apr- 2020].

[101] "Scientific Opinion on the substantiation of health claims related to vitamin B6", *Efsa.onlinelibrary.wiley.com*, 2010. [Online]. Available: https://efsa.onlinelibrary.wiley.com/doi/epdf/10.2903/j.efsa.2010.1759. [Accessed: 12- Apr- 2020].

[102] M. Davidson, "Molecular Expressions: The Vitamin Collection - Pyridoxine (Pyridoxal phosphate, Vitamin B-6)", *Micro.magnet.fsu.edu*, 2018. [Online]. Available: https://micro.magnet.fsu.edu/vitamins/pages/pyridoxine.html. [Accessed: 31- May- 2020].

[103] "Office of Dietary Supplements - Vitamin B6", *Ods.od.nih.gov*, 2020. [Online]. Available: https://ods.od.nih.gov/factsheets/VitaminB6-HealthProfessional/. [Accessed: 30- Apr- 2020].

[104] "Scientific Opinion on the substantiation of health claims related to vitamin B12", *Efsa.onlinelibrary.wiley.com*, 2010. [Online]. Available: https://efsa.onlinelibrary.wiley.com/doi/epdf/10.2903/j.efsa.2010.1756. [Accessed: 12- Apr- 2020].

[105] "The discovery of Pernicious anaemia", *ari.info*, 2014. [Online]. Available: http://www.animalresearch.info/en/medical-advances/timeline/pernicious-anaemia/. [Accessed: 31- May- 2020].

[106] "Office of Dietary Supplements - Vitamin B12", *Ods.od.nih.gov*, 2020. [Online]. Available: https://ods.od.nih.gov/factsheets/VitaminB12-HealthProfessional/. [Accessed: 30- Apr- 2020].

[107] F. Callaghan, K. Leishear, S. Abhyankar, D. Demner-Fushman and C. McDonald, "High vitamin B12 levels are not associated with increased mortality risk for ICU patients after adjusting for liver function: A cohort study", *e-SPEN Journal*, vol. 9, no. 2, pp. e76-e83, 2014. Available: https://www.ncbi.nlm.nih.gov/pmc/articles/PMC3961712/. [Accessed 11 May 2020].

[108] "The Baobab Tree:Africa's Iconic "Tree of Life"", *Aduna*, 2020. [Online]. Available: https://aduna.com/blogs/learn/the-baobab-tree. [Accessed: 31- May- 2020].

[109] M. Petruzzello, "baobab | Description, Species, Distribution, & Importance", *Encyclopedia Britannica*, 2018. [Online]. Available: https://www.britannica.com/plant/baobab-tree-genus. [Accessed: 30- Apr- 2020].

[110] A. Zarei, S. Changizi-Ashtiyani, S. Taheri and M. Ramezani, "A quick overview on some aspects of endocrinological and therapeutic effects of Berberis vulgaris L.", *Europepmc.org*, 2015. [Online]. Available: https://europepmc.org/backend/ptpmcrender.fcgi?accid=PMC4678494&blobtype=pdf. [Accessed: 31- May- 2020].

[111] "National Center for Biotechnology Information. PubChem Database. Berberine, CID=2353", *Pubchem.ncbi.nlm.nih.gov*, 2020. [Online]. Available: https://pubchem.ncbi.nlm.nih.gov/compound/2353. [Accessed: 12- Apr- 2020].

[112] M. Siervo, J. Lara, I. Ogbonmwan and J. Mathers, "Inorganic Nitrate and Beetroot Juice Supplementation Reduces Blood Pressure in Adults: A Systematic Review and Meta-Analysis", *The Journal of Nutrition*, vol. 143, no. 6, pp. 818-826, 2013. Available: https://academic.oup.com/jn/article/143/6/818/4571708. [Accessed 12 April 2020].

[113] "Berberine: MedlinePlus Supplements", *Medlineplus.gov*, 2019. [Online]. Available: https://medlineplus.gov/druginfo/natural/1126.html. [Accessed: 15- May- 2020].

[114] A. DuPont, D. Richards, K. Jelinek, J. Krill, E. Rahimi and Y. Ghouri, "Systematic review of randomized controlled trials of probiotics, prebiotics, and synbiotics in inflammatory bowel disease", *Clinical and Experimental Gastroenterology*, p. 473, 2014. Available: https://pubmed.ncbi.nlm.nih.gov/25525379/. [Accessed 12 April 2020].

[115] M. Schell et al., "The genome sequence of Bifidobacterium longum reflects its adaptation to the human gastrointestinal tract", *Proceedings of the National Academy of Sciences*, vol. 99, no. 22, pp. 14422-14427, 2002. Available: https://www.pnas.org/content/99/22/14422. [Accessed 30 April 2020].

[116] "Bifidobacteria: MedlinePlus Supplements", *Medlineplus.gov*, 2019. [Online]. Available: https://medlineplus.gov/druginfo/natural/891.html. [Accessed: 26- May- 2020].

[117] W. Chu, S. Cheung, R. Lau and I. Benzie, "Bilberry (Vaccinium myrtillus L.)", *Ncbi.nlm.nih.gov*, 2011. [Online]. Available: https://www.ncbi.nlm.nih.gov/books/NBK92770/. [Accessed: 12- Apr- 2020].

[118] *Nccih.nih.gov*, 2016. [Online]. Available: https://www.nccih.nih.gov/health/bilberry [Accessed: 21- May- 2020].

[119] "Scientific Opinion on the substantiation of health claims related to biotin", *Efsa.onlinelibrary.wiley.com*, 2010. [Online]. Available: https://efsa.onlinelibrary.wiley.com/doi/epdf/10.2903/j.efsa.2010.1728. [Accessed: 12- Apr- 2020].

[120] "Office of Dietary Supplements - Biotin", *Ods.od.nih.gov*, 2017. [Online]. Available: https://ods.od.nih.gov/factsheets/Biotin-Consumer/. [Accessed: 21- May- 2020].

[121] "Vitamins and minerals - B vitamins and folic acid", *nhs.uk*, 2020. [Online]. Available: https://www.nhs.uk/conditions/vitamins-and-minerals/vitamin-b/. [Accessed: 12- Apr- 2020].

[122] "Office of Dietary Supplements - Biotin", *Ods.od.nih.gov*, 2020. [Online]. Available: https://ods.od.nih.gov/factsheets/Biotin-HealthProfessional/. [Accessed: 30- Apr- 2020].

[123] *Nccih.nih.gov*, 2019. [Online]. Available: https://www.nccih.nih.gov/health/bitter-

orange. [Accessed: 22- May- 2020].

[124] A. Gopalan, S. Reuben, S. Ahmed, A. Darvesh, J. Hohmann and A. Bishayee, "The health benefits of blackcurrants", *Food & Function*, vol. 3, no. 8, p. 795, 2012. Available: https://pubmed.ncbi.nlm.nih.gov/22673662/. [Accessed 30 April 2020].

[125] H. Traitler, H. Winter, U. Richli and Y. Ingenbleek, "Characterization of γ-linolenic acid inRibes seed", *Lipids*, vol. 19, no. 12, pp. 923-928, 1984. Available: https://pubmed.ncbi.nlm.nih.gov/6098796/. [Accessed 30 April 2020].

[126] "Office of Dietary Supplements - Black Cohosh", Ods.od.nih.gov, 2020. [Online]. Available: https://ods.od.nih.gov/factsheets/BlackCohosh-HealthProfessional/. [Accessed: 04- May- 2020].

[127] G. Saravanan and P. Ponmurugan, "S-allylcysteine Improves Streptozotocin-Induced Alterations of Blood Glucose, Liver Cytochrome P450 2E1, Plasma Antioxidant System, and Adipocytes Hormones in Diabetic Rats", *International Journal of Endocrinology and Metabolism*, vol. 11, no. 4, 2013. Available: https://www.ncbi.nlm.nih.gov/pmc/articles/PMC3968993/. [Accessed 12 April 2020].

[128] A. Colín-González, S. Ali, I. Túnez and A. Santamaría, "On the antioxidant, neuroprotective and anti-inflammatory properties of S-allyl cysteine: An update", *Neurochemistry International*, vol. 89, pp. 83-91, 2015. Available: https://www.sciencedirect.com/science/article/abs/pii/S0197018615000959. [Accessed 12 April 2020].

[129] Melissa, "A Brief History of Pepper", *Today I Found Out*, 2020. [Online]. Available: http://www.todayifoundout.com/index.php/2014/01/brief-history-pepper/. [Accessed: 31- May- 2020].

[130] S. Mishra and K. Palanivelu, "The effect of curcumin (turmeric) onAlzheimer's disease: An overview", *Annals of Indian Academy of Neurology*, vol. 11, no. 1, p. 13, 2008. Available: https://www.ncbi.nlm.nih.gov/pmc/articles/PMC2781139/. [Accessed 12 April 2020].

[131] "Black Tea: MedlinePlus Supplements", *Medlineplus.gov*, 2019. [Online]. Available: https://medlineplus.gov/druginfo/natural/997.html. [Accessed: 15- May- 2020].

[132] "Epidemiology | Definition of Epidemiology by Lexico", *Lexico Dictionaries | English*, 2020. [Online]. Available: https://www.lexico.com/en/definition/epidemiology. [Accessed: 31- May- 2020].

[133] W. Kalt et al., "Recent Research on the Health Benefits of Blueberries and Their Anthocyanins", *Advances in Nutrition*, 2019. Available: https://academic.oup.com/advances/article/11/2/224/5536953. [Accessed 31 May 2020].

[134] G. Logan, "Foodie Guide to Borragine", *ITALY Magazine*, 2012. [Online]. Available: https://www.italymagazine.com/featured-story/foodie-guide-borragine. [Accessed: 21- Jun- 2020].

[135] A. Gilani, S. Bashir and A. Khan, "Pharmacological basis for the use of Borago officinalis in gastrointestinal, respiratory and cardiovascular disorders", *Journal of Ethnopharmacology*,

vol. 114, no. 3, pp. 393-399, 2007. Available: https://pubmed.ncbi.nlm.nih.gov/17900837/. [Accessed 21 June 2020].

[136] "Borage seed oil", *Versus Arthritis*, 2018. [Online]. Available: https://www.versusarthritis.org/about-arthritis/complementary-and-alternative-treatments/types-of-complementary-treatments/borage-seed-oil/. [Accessed: 21- Jun- 2020].

[137] C. Dodson and F. Stermitz, "Pyrrolizidine Alkaloids from Borage (Borago officinalis) Seeds and Flowers", *Journal of Natural Products*, vol. 49, no. 4, pp. 727-728, 1986. Available: https://pubs.acs.org/doi/abs/10.1021/np50046a045. [Accessed 21 June 2020].

[138] P. Buck, "Origin and taxonomy of broccoli", *Economic Botany*, vol. 10, no. 3, pp. 250-253, 1956. Available: https://link.springer.com/article/10.1007%2FBF02899000. [Accessed 15 May 2020].

[139] "Broccoli | Meaning of Broccoli by Lexico", *Lexico Dictionaries* | English, 2020. [Online]. Available: https://www.lexico.com/definition/broccoli. [Accessed: 22- May- 2020].

[140] "Broccus word origin", Etymologeek, 2020. [Online]. Available: https://etymologeek.com/lat/broccus. [Accessed: 22- May- 2020].

[141] *Nccih.nih.gov*, 2016. [Online]. Available: https://www.nccih.nih.gov/health/butterbur. [Accessed: 22- Apr- 2020].

[142] A. Rapoport, *Americanheadachesociety.org*. [Online]. Available: https://americanheadachesociety.org/wp-content/uploads/2018/05/Alan_Rapoport_-_Migraine_Prevention_Medications.pdf. [Accessed: 22- May- 2020].

[143] A. Hume, *Pharmacytoday.org*, 2019. [Online]. Available: https://www.pharmacytoday.org/article/S1042-0991(19)30366-4/pdf. [Accessed: 22- May- 2020].

[144] T. P, L. B, C. B, K. C and H. C, "Ragweed (Ambrosia) progression and its health risks: will Switzerland resist this invasion?", PubMed, 2022. [Online]. Available: https://pubmed.ncbi.nlm.nih.gov/16333764/. [Accessed: 03- Jan- 2022].

[145] H. Hemilä and E. Chalker, "Vitamin C for preventing and treating the common cold", *Cochrane Database of Systematic Reviews*, 2013. Available: https://www.cochranelibrary.com/cdsr/doi/10.1002/14651858.CD000980.pub4/epdf/standard. [Accessed 13 April 2020].

[146] G. Drouin, J. Godin and B. Page, "The Genetics of Vitamin C Loss in Vertebrates", *Current Genomics*, vol. 12, no. 5, pp. 371-378, 2011. Available: https://www.ncbi.nlm.nih.gov/pmc/articles/PMC3145266/. [Accessed 1 June 2020].

[147] "Vitamins and minerals - Vitamin C", *nhs.uk*, 2020. [Online]. Available: https://www.nhs.uk/conditions/vitamins-and-minerals/vitamin-c/. [Accessed: 21- May- 2020].

[148] "Scientific Opinion on the substantiation of health claims related to vitamin C", *Efsa.onlinelibrary.wiley.com*, 2009. [Online]. Available: https://efsa.onlinelibrary.wiley.com/doi/epdf/10.2903/j.efsa.2009.1226. [Accessed: 13- Apr- 2020].

[149] "Office of Dietary Supplements - Vitamin C", *Ods.od.nih.gov*, 2020. [Online]. Available: https://ods.od.nih.gov/factsheets/VitaminC-HealthProfessional/. [Accessed: 01- May- 2020].

[150] A. Carr and B. Frei, "Toward a new recommended dietary allowance for vitamin C based on antioxidant and health effects in humans", *The American Journal of Clinical Nutrition*, vol. 69, no. 6, pp. 1086-1107, 1999. Available: https://academic.oup.com/ajcn/article/69/6/1086/4714888. [Accessed 1 May 2020].

[151] *Sheffield.ac.uk*. [Online]. Available: https://www.sheffield.ac.uk/FRAX/tool.aspx?country=1. [Accessed: 30- Apr- 2021].

[152] "Office of Dietary Supplements - Calcium", *Ods.od.nih.gov*, 2020. [Online]. Available: https://ods.od.nih.gov/factsheets/Calcium-HealthProfessional/. [Accessed: 31- Apr- 2020].

[153] A. Ross, C. Taylor, A. Yaktine and H. Valle, "Tolerable Upper Intake Levels: Calcium and Vitamin D", *Ncbi.nlm.nih.gov*, 2011. [Online]. Available: https://www.ncbi.nlm.nih.gov/books/NBK56058/. [Accessed: 11- May- 2020].

[154] J. Elliott et al., "Cannabis-based products for pediatric epilepsy: An updated systematic review", *Seizure*, vol. 75, pp. 18-22, 2020. Available: https://pubmed.ncbi.nlm.nih.gov/31865133/. [Accessed 15 May 2020].

[155] B. Dykes, "World's hottest pepper is 'hot enough to strip paint'", *News.yahoo.com*, 2010. [Online]. Available: https://news.yahoo.com/blogs/lookout/world-hottest-pepper-hot-enough-strip-paint.html. [Accessed: 01- Jun- 2020].

[156] B. Hallcock, "World's hottest pepper hits 2.2 million Scoville heat units", *Los Angeles Times*, 2013. [Online]. Available: https://www.latimes.com/food/dailydish/la-dd-worlds-hottest-pepper-scoville-heat-units-20131226-story.html. [Accessed: 01- Jun- 2020].

[157] J. Tewksbury, "NPR Choice page",*Npr.org*, 2008. [Online]. Available: https://www.npr.org/templates/story/story.php?storyId=93636630&t=1591007567135. [Accessed: 01- Jun- 2020].

[158] "Scientific Opinion on the substantiation of health claims related to capsaicin and maintenance of body weight after weight loss", *Efsa.onlinelibrary.wiley.com*, 2011. [Online]. Available: https://efsa.onlinelibrary.wiley.com/doi/epdf/10.2903/j.efsa.2011.2210. [Accessed: 13- May- 2020].

[159] "Capsicum: MedlinePlus Supplements", *Medlineplus.gov*, 2019. [Online]. Available: https://medlineplus.gov/druginfo/natural/945.html. [Accessed: 11- May- 2020].

[160] E. Leoncini, D. Nedovic, N. Panic, R. Pastorino, V. Edefonti and S. Boccia, "Carotenoid Intake from Natural Sources and Head and Neck Cancer: A Systematic Review and Meta-analysis of Epidemiological Studies", *Cancer Epidemiology Biomarkers & Prevention*, vol. 24, no. 7, pp. 1003-1011, 2015. Available: https://pubmed.ncbi.nlm.nih.gov/25873578/. [Accessed 25 April 2020].

[161] C. Soares, A. Teodoro, P. Lotsch, J. Granjeiro and R. Borojevic, "Anticancer Properties of Carotenoids in Prostate Cancer. A Review", *PubMed*, 2015. [Online]. Available: https://pubmed.ncbi.nlm.nih.gov/26058846/. [Accessed: 25- Apr- 2020].

[162] S. Schagen, V. Zampeli, E. Makrantonaki and C. Zouboulis, "Discovering the link be-

tween nutrition and skin aging", *Dermato-Endocrinology*, vol. 4, no. 3, pp. 298-307, 2012. Available: https://pubmed.ncbi.nlm.nih.gov/23467449/. [Accessed 25 April 2020].

[163] C. Lizarazo, A. Lampi, P. Mäkelä and J. Leppälä, "Finnish caraway: is place of cultivation critical for high quality? | Request PDF", *ResearchGate*, 2019. [Online]. Available: https://www.researchgate.net/publication/333609661_Finnish_caraway_is_place_of_cultivation_critical_for_high_quality. [Accessed: 01- Jun- 2020].

[164] Y. Zheng et al., "The laxative effect of emodin is attributable to increased aquaporin 3 expression in the colon of mice and HT-29 cells", *Fitoterapia*, vol. 96, pp. 25-32, 2014. Available: https://doi.org/10.1016/j.fitote.2014.04.002. [Accessed 26 May 2020].

[165] A. Primeau, "Cascara and Cancer - Cancer Therapy Advisor", *Cancer Therapy Advisor*, 2018. [Online]. Available: https://www.cancertherapyadvisor.com/home/tools/factsheets/cascara-and-cancer/2/. [Accessed: 26- May- 2020].

[166] "American Botanical Council: The ABC Clinical Guide to Herbs", *Cms.herbalgram.org*. [Online]. Available: http://cms.herbalgram.org/ABCGuide/Monographs/CatsClaw.html. [Accessed: 26- May- 2020].

[167] *Nccih.nih.gov*, 2016. [Online]. Available: https://www.nccih.nih.gov/health/cats-claw. [Accessed: 26- May- 2020].

[168] "Interesting facts about cauliflower | Just Fun Facts", *Justfunfacts.com*, 2018. [Online]. Available: http://justfunfacts.com/interesting-facts-about-cauliflower/. [Accessed: 01- Jun- 2020].

[169] *Nccih.nih.gov*, 2016. [Online]. Available: https://www.nccih.nih.gov/health/chamomile. [Accessed: 23- May- 2020].

[170] D. McKay and J. Blumberg, "A Review of the bioactivity and potential health benefits of chamomile tea (Matricaria recutita L.)", *Phytotherapy Research*, vol. 20, no. 7, pp. 519-530, 2006. Available: https://pubmed.ncbi.nlm.nih.gov/16628544/. [Accessed 27 April 2020].

[171] F. Hajizadeh-Sharafabad, P. Varshosaz, H. Jafari-Vayghan, M. Alizadeh and V. Maleki, "Chamomile (Matricaria recutita L.) and diabetes mellitus, current knowledge and the way forward: A systematic review", *Complementary Therapies in Medicine*, vol. 48, p. 102284, 2020. Available: https://www.sciencedirect.com/science/article/pii/S096522991930901X. [Accessed 23 May 2020].

[172] "Chicory greens, raw", 2020. [Online]. Available: https://fdc.nal.usda.gov/fdc-app.html#/food-details/169992/nutrients. [Accessed: 27- Apr- 2021].

[173] "The History of Coffee & Chicory", *Communitycoffee.com*, 2020. [Online]. Available: https://www.communitycoffee.com/blog/detail/the-history-of-coffee-chicory. [Accessed: 27- May- 2020].

[174] "Fact sheet about Malaria", *Who.int*, 2020. [Online]. Available: https://www.who.int/news-room/fact-sheets/detail/malaria. [Accessed: 14- May- 2020].

[175] S. Gu and J. Pei, "Innovating Chinese Herbal Medicine: From Traditional Health Practice to Scientific Drug Discovery", *Frontiers in Pharmacology*, vol. 8, 2017. Available: https://www.ncbi.nlm.nih.gov/pmc/articles/PMC5472722/. [Accessed 14 May 2020].

[176] A. Bode and Z. Dong, "The Amazing and Mighty Ginger", *Ncbi.nlm.nih.gov*, 2011. [Online]. Available: https://www.ncbi.nlm.nih.gov/books/NBK92775/. [Accessed: 14- May- 2020].

[177] G. Thompson, A. Husney MD and M. Gabica, "Chloride (Cl) | Michigan Medicine", *Uofmhealth.org*, 2019. [Online]. Available: https://www.uofmhealth.org/health-library/hw6323. [Accessed: 27- Apr- 2020].

[178] H. Zhu, C. Hart, D. Sales and N. Roberts, "Bacterial killing in gastric juice – effect of pH and pepsin on Escherichia coli and Helicobacter pylori", *Journal of Medical Microbiology*, vol. 55, no. 9, pp. 1265-1270, 2006. Available: https://pubmed.ncbi.nlm.nih.gov/16914658/. [Accessed 27 April 2020].

[179] S. Zeisel, "A Brief History of Choline", *Annals of Nutrition and Metabolism*, vol. 61, no. 3, pp. 254-258, 2012. Available: https://www.ncbi.nlm.nih.gov/pmc/articles/PMC4422379/. [Accessed 1 June 2020].

[180] "Scientific Opinion on the substantiation of health claims related to choline", *Efsa.onlinelibrary.wiley.com*, 2011. [Online]. Available: https://efsa.onlinelibrary.wiley.com/doi/epdf/10.2903/j.efsa.2011.2056. [Accessed: 13- Apr- 2020].

[181] "Office of Dietary Supplements - Choline", *Ods.od.nih.gov*, 2020. [Online]. Available: https://ods.od.nih.gov/factsheets/Choline-HealthProfessional/. [Accessed: 30- Apr- 2020].

[182] "Office of Dietary Supplements - Dietary Supplement Fact Sheet: Chromium", *Ods.od.nih.gov*, 2020. [Online]. Available: https://ods.od.nih.gov/factsheets/Chromium-HealthProfessional/#h3. [Accessed: 30- Apr- 2020].

[183] "Cinquefoil | plant", *Encyclopedia Britannica*, 2020. [Online]. Available: https://www.britannica.com/plant/cinquefoil. [Accessed: 01- Jun- 2020].

[184] R. Huber et al., "Tormentil for Active Ulcerative Colitis", *Journal of Clinical Gastroenterology*, vol. 41, no. 9, pp. 834-838, 2007. Available: https://pubmed.ncbi.nlm.nih.gov/17881930/. [Accessed 27 April 2020].

[185] M. Leach and S. Kumar, "Cinnamon for diabetes mellitus", *Cochrane Database of Systematic Reviews*, 2012. Available: https://www.cochranelibrary.com/cdsr/doi/10.1002/14651858.CD007170.pub2/abstract. [Accessed 23 May 2020].

[186] A. Mbaveng and V. Kuete, "Syzygium aromaticum - an overview | ScienceDirect Topics", *Sciencedirect.com*, 2017. [Online]. Available: https://www.sciencedirect.com/topics/agricultural-and-biological-sciences/syzygium-aromaticum. [Accessed: 26- May- 2020].

[187] "Cobalt - Health Encyclopedia - University of Rochester Medical Center", *Urmc.rochester.edu*, 2020. [Online]. Available: https://www.urmc.rochester.edu/encyclopedia/content.aspx?contenttypeid=19&contentid=Cobalt. [Accessed: 01- May- 2020].

[188] *Nccih.nih.gov*, 2019. [Online]. Available: https://www.nccih.nih.gov/health/coenzyme-

q10. [Accessed: 15- May- 2020].

[189] W. Judy, W. Stogsdill and K. Folkers, "Myocardial preservation by therapy with coenzyme Q10 during heart surgery", *The Clinical Investigator*, vol. 71, no. 8, 1993. Available: https://pubmed.ncbi.nlm.nih.gov/8241702/. [Accessed 15 May 2020].

[190] R. Wapnir and C. Balkman, "Inhibition of copper absorption by zinc", *Biological Trace Element Research*, vol. 29, no. 3, pp. 193-202, 1991. Available: https://pubmed.ncbi.nlm.nih.gov/1726403/. [Accessed 27 April 2020].

[191] "Office of Dietary Supplements - Copper", *Ods.od.nih.gov*, 2020. [Online]. Available: https://ods.od.nih.gov/factsheets/Copper-HealthProfessional/. [Accessed: 27- Apr- 2020].

[192] R. Jepson, G. Williams and J. Craig, "Cranberries for preventing urinary tract infections", *Cochrane Database of Systematic Reviews*, 2012. Available: https://www.cochranelibrary.com/cdsr/doi/10.1002/14651858.CD001321.pub5/abstract. [Accessed 22 July 2020].

[193] "Curcumin and normal functioning of joints", *Efsa.onlinelibrary.wiley.com*, 2017. [Online]. Available: https://efsa.onlinelibrary.wiley.com/doi/epdf/10.2903/j.efsa.2017.4774. [Accessed: 13- Apr- 2020].

[194] S. Hewlings and D. Kalman, "Curcumin: A Review of Its' Effects on Human Health", *Foods*, vol. 6, no. 10, p. 92, 2017. Available: https://www.ncbi.nlm.nih.gov/pmc/articles/PMC5664031/. [Accessed 23 April 2020].

[195] A. Pompella, A. Visvikis, A. Paolicchi, V. Tata and A. Casini, "The changing faces of glutathione, a cellular protagonist", *Biochemical Pharmacology*, vol. 66, no. 8, pp. 1499-1503, 2003. Available: https://www.sciencedirect.com/science/article/abs/pii/S0006295203005045. [Accessed 12 May 2021].

[196] B. Dawson-Hughes, S. Harris, A. Lichtenstein, G. Dolnikowski, N. Palermo and H. Rasmussen, "Dietary Fat Increases Vitamin D-3 Absorption", *Journal of the Academy of Nutrition and Dietetics*, vol. 115, no. 2, pp. 225-230, 2015. Available: https://pubmed.ncbi.nlm.nih.gov/25441954/. [Accessed 14 April 2020].

[197] K. Cashman et al., "Vitamin D deficiency in Europe: pandemic?", *The American Journal of Clinical Nutrition*, vol. 103, no. 4, pp. 1033-1044, 2016. Available: https://academic.oup.com/ajcn/article/103/4/1033/4662891. [Accessed 15 April 2020].

[198] M. Melamed, E. Michos, W. Post and B. Astor, "25-Hydroxyvitamin D Levels and the Risk of Mortality in the General Population", *Archives of Internal Medicine*, vol. 168, no. 15, pp. 1629-1637, 2008. Available: https://jamanetwork.com/journals/jamainternalmedicine/fullarticle/770360. [Accessed 15 April 2020].

[199] L. Black, R. Lucas, J. Sherriff, L. Björn and J. Bornman, "In Pursuit of Vitamin D in Plants", *Nutrients*, vol. 9, no. 2, p. 136, 2017. Available: https://www.ncbi.nlm.nih.gov/pmc/articles/PMC5331567/. [Accessed 15 April 2020].

[200] J. Pittaway, K. Ahuja, J. Beckett, M. Bird, I. Robertson and M. Ball, "Make Vitamin D While

the Sun Shines, Take Supplements When It Doesn't: A Longitudinal, Observational Study of Older Adults in Tasmania, Australia", *PLoS ONE*, vol. 8, no. 3, p. e59063, 2013. Available: https://journals.plos.org/plosone/article?id=10.1371/journal.pone.0059063. [Accessed 2 June 2020].

[201] "Vitamins and minerals - Vitamin D", *nhs.uk*, 2017. [Online]. Available: https://www.nhs.uk/conditions/vitamins-and-minerals/vitamin-d/. [Accessed: 15- Apr- 2020].

[202] V. Mehta and S. Agarwal, "Does Vitamin D Deficiency Lead to Hypertension?", *Cureus*, 2017. Available: https://www.ncbi.nlm.nih.gov/pmc/articles/PMC5356990/. [Accessed 16 April 2020].

[203] "Taking too much vitamin D can cloud its benefits and create health risks - Harvard Health", *Harvard Health*, 2017. [Online]. Available: https://www.health.harvard.edu/staying-healthy/taking-too-much-vitamin-d-can-cloud-its-benefits-and-create-health-risks. [Accessed: 15- Apr- 2020].

[204] "Office of Dietary Supplements - Vitamin D", *Ods.od.nih.gov*, 2020. [Online]. Available: https://ods.od.nih.gov/factsheets/VitaminD-HealthProfessional/. [Accessed: 30- Apr- 2020].

[205] H. Zhu et al., "Dandelion root extract suppressed gastric cancer cells proliferation and migration through targeting lncRNA-CCAT1", *Biomedicine & Pharmacotherapy*, vol. 93, pp. 1010-1017, 2017. Available: https://www.sciencedirect.com/science/article/pii/S075333221731987X. [Accessed 13 April 2020].

[206] "Dandelion greens, raw Nutrition Facts & Calories", *Nutritiondata.self.com*, 2018. [Online]. Available: https://nutritiondata.self.com/facts/vegetables-and-vegetable-products/2441/2. [Accessed: 01- May- 2020].

[207] T. Huang et al., "Harpagoside suppresses lipopolysaccharide-induced iNOS and COX-2 expression through inhibition of NF-κB activation", *Journal of Ethnopharmacology*, vol. 104, no. 1-2, pp. 149-155, 2006. Available: https://pubmed.ncbi.nlm.nih.gov/16203115/. [Accessed 16 April 2020].

[208] "Harpagophyti radix - European Medicines Agency", *European Medicines Agency*, 2016. [Online]. Available: https://www.ema.europa.eu/en/medicines/herbal/harpagophyti-radix. [Accessed: 02- Jun- 2020].

[209] T. Conrozier et al,, "A Complex of Three Natural Anti-Inflammatory Agents Provides Relief of Osteoarthritis Pain", *PubMed*, 2014. [Online]. Available: https://pubmed.ncbi.nlm.nih.gov/24473984/. [Accessed: 16- May- 2020].

[210] J. Bradbury, "Docosahexaenoic Acid (DHA): An Ancient Nutrient for the Modern Human Brain", *Nutrients*, vol. 3, no. 5, pp. 529-554, 2011. Available: https://www.ncbi.nlm.nih.gov/pmc/articles/PMC3257695/. [Accessed 30 April 2020].

[211] P. Saravanan, N. Davidson, E. Schmidt and P. Calder, "Cardiovascular effects of marine omega-3 fatty acids", *The Lancet*, vol. 376, no. 9740, pp. 540-550, 2010. Available: https://pubmed.ncbi.nlm.nih.gov/20638121/. [Accessed 30 April 2020].

[212] L. Horrocks and Y. Yeo, "Health benefits of Docosahexaenoic Acid (DHA)",

Pharmacological Research, vol. 40, no. 3, pp. 211-225, 1999. Available: https://pubmed.ncbi.nlm.nih.gov/10479465/. [Accessed 13 April 2020].

[213] H. Evans and K. Bishop, "On the Existence of a Hitherto Unrecognized Dietary Factor Essential for Reproduction", *Science*, vol. 56, no. 1458, pp. 650-651, 1922. Available: https://science.sciencemag.org/content/56/1458/650. [Accessed 3 June 2020].

[214] E. Oakes, "Encyclopedia of World Scientists", *Google Books*, 2007. [Online]. Available: https://books.google.co.uk/books?id=uPRB-OED1bcC&pg=PA211&redir_esc=y#v=onepage&q&f=false. [Accessed: 03- Jun- 2020].

[215] "Scientific Opinion on the substantiation of health claims related to vitamin E", *Efsa.onlinelibrary.wiley.com*, 2010. [Online]. Available: https://efsa.onlinelibrary.wiley.com/doi/epdf/10.2903/j.efsa.2010.1816. [Accessed: 17- Apr- 2020].

[216] "Vitamins and minerals - Vitamin E", *nhs.uk*, 2017. [Online]. Available: https://www.nhs.uk/conditions/vitamins-and-minerals/vitamin-e/. [Accessed: 17- Apr- 2020].

[217] "Office of Dietary Supplements - Vitamin E", *Ods.od.nih.gov*, 2020. [Online]. Available: https://ods.od.nih.gov/factsheets/VitaminE-HealthProfessional/. [Accessed: 30- Apr- 2020].

[218] *Nccih.nih.gov*, 2016. [Online]. Available: https://www.nccih.nih.gov/health/echinacea. [Accessed: 15- May- 2020].

[219] "Ellagic Acid - an overview | ScienceDirect Topics", *Sciencedirect.com*, 2017. [Online]. Available: https://www.sciencedirect.com/topics/medicine-and-dentistry/ellagic-acid. [Accessed: 13- Apr- 2020].

[220] W. Chen et al., "A Review: The Bioactivities and Pharmacological Applications of Phellinus linteus", *Molecules*, vol. 24, no. 10, p. 1888, 2019. Available: https://www.mdpi.com/1420-3049/24/10/1888. [Accessed 3 June 2020].

[221] S. Weng, J. Tang, G. Wang, X. Wang and H. Wang, "Comparison of the Addition of Siberian Ginseng (Acanthopanax senticosus) Versus Fluoxetine to Lithium for the Treatment of Bipolar Disorder in Adolescents: A Randomized, Double-Blind Trial", *Current Therapeutic Research*, vol. 68, no. 4, pp. 280-290, 2007. Available: https://www.ncbi.nlm.nih.gov/pmc/articles/PMC3967289/. [Accessed 16 May 2020].

[222] E. Freye and J. Gleske, "Siberian Ginseng Results in Beneficial Effects on Glucose Metabolism in Diabetes Type 2 Patients: A Double Blind Placebo-Controlled Study in Comparison to Panax Ginseng", *Pubs.sciepub.com*, 2013. [Online]. Available: http://pubs.sciepub.com/ijcn/1/1/2/. [Accessed: 03- Jun- 2020].

[223] S. Ehrlich, "Complementary and Alternative Medicine - Penn State Hershey Medical Center - Siberian ginseng - Penn State Hershey Medical Center", *Pennstatehershey.adam.com*, 2015. [Online]. Available: http://pennstatehershey.adam.com/content.aspx?productid=107&pid=33&gid=000250. [Accessed: 03- Jun- 2020].

[224] G. H, "Can Adults Adequately Convert Alpha-Linolenic Acid (18:3n-3) to Eicosapentaenoic Acid (20:5n-3) and Docosahexaenoic Acid (22:6n-3)?", *PubMed*, 1998. [Online]. Available:

https://pubmed.ncbi.nlm.nih.gov/9637947/. [Accessed: 03- Jun- 2020].

[225] Nccih.nih.gov, 2016. [Online]. Available: https://www.nccih.nih.gov/health/european-elder. [Accessed: 15- May- 2020].

[226] M. May, "Is Mistletoe Poisonous?", *Poison.org*. [Online]. Available: https://www.poison.org/articles/2015-dec/mistletoe. [Accessed: 23- May- 2020].

[227] "Mistletoe Extracts (PDQ®)–Patient Version", *National Cancer Institute*. [Online]. Available: https://www.cancer.gov/about-cancer/treatment/cam/patient/mistletoe-pdq. [Accessed: 03- Jun- 2020].

[228] P. Mansky et al., "NCCAM/NCI Phase 1 Study of Mistletoe Extract and Gemcitabine in Patients with Advanced Solid Tumors", *Evidence-Based Complementary and Alternative Medicine*, vol. 2013, pp. 1-11, 2013. Available: https://pubmed.ncbi.nlm.nih.gov/24285980/. [Accessed 3 June 2020].

[229] *Nccih.nih.gov*, 2016. [Online]. Available: https://www.nccih.nih.gov/health/evening-primrose-oil. [Accessed: 28- Apr- 2020].

[230] S. Badgujar, V. Patel and A. Bandivdekar, "Foeniculum vulgareMill: A Review of Its Botany, Phytochemistry, Pharmacology, Contemporary Application, and Toxicology", *BioMed Research International*, vol. 2014, pp. 1-32, 2014. Available: https://www.ncbi.nlm.nih.gov/pmc/articles/PMC4137549/. [Accessed 3 June 2020].

[231] "Tanacetum parthenium | feverfew/RHS Gardening", *Rhs.org.uk*. [Online]. Available: https://www.rhs.org.uk/Plants/17986/i-Tanacetum-parthenium-i/Details. [Accessed: 27- Apr- 2020].

[232] A. Pareek, M. Suthar, G. Rathore and V. Bansal, "Feverfew (Tanacetum parthenium L.): A systematic review", *Pharmacognosy Reviews*, vol. 5, no. 9, p. 103, 2011. Available: https://www.ncbi.nlm.nih.gov/pmc/articles/PMC3210009/. [Accessed 27 April 2020].

[233] D. Davani-Davari et al., "Prebiotics: Definition, Types, Sources, Mechanisms, and Clinical Applications", *Foods*, vol. 8, no. 3, p. 92, 2019. Available: https://www.ncbi.nlm.nih.gov/pmc/articles/PMC6463098/. [Accessed 5 May 2020].

[234] M. Eastwood and D. Kritchevsky, "DIETARY FIBER: How Did We Get Where We Are?", *Annual Review of Nutrition*, vol. 25, no. 1, pp. 1-8, 2005. Available: https://pubmed.ncbi.nlm.nih.gov/16011456/. [Accessed 5 May 2020].

[235] A. Reynolds, J. Mann, J. Cummings, N. Winter, E. Mete and L. Te Morenga, "Carbohydrate quality and human health: a series of systematic reviews and meta-analyses", *The Lancet*, vol. 393, no. 10170, pp. 434-445, 2019. Available: https://pubmed.ncbi.nlm.nih.gov/30638909/. [Accessed 5 May 2020].

[236] Y. Park, A. Subar, A. Hollenbeck and A. Schatzkin, "Dietary Fiber Intake and Mortality in the NIH-AARP Diet and Health Study", *Archives of Internal Medicine*, vol. 171, no. 12, 2011. Available: https://pubmed.ncbi.nlm.nih.gov/21321288/. [Accessed 5 May 2020].

[237] "How to get more fibre into your diet", *nhs.uk*, 2018. [Online]. Available: https://

www.nhs.uk/live-well/eat-well/how-to-get-more-fibre-into-your-diet/. [Accessed: 07- May- 2020].

[238] A. Goyal, V. Sharma, N. Upadhyay, S. Gill and M. Sihag, "Flax and flaxseed oil: an ancient medicine & modern functional food", *Journal of Food Science and Technology*, vol. 51, no. 9, pp. 1633-1653, 2014. Available: https://www.ncbi.nlm.nih.gov/pmc/articles/PMC4152533/. [Accessed 3 June 2020].

[239] *Who.int*, 2004. [Online]. Available: https://www.who.int/water_sanitation_health/dwq/chemicals/fluoride.pdf. [Accessed: 27- Apr- 2020].

[240] M. Aarabi et al., "High-dose folic acid supplementation alters the human sperm methylome and is influenced by theMTHFRC677T polymorphism", *Human Molecular Genetics*, vol. 24, no. 22, pp. 6301-6313, 2015. Available: https://pubmed.ncbi.nlm.nih.gov/26307085/. [Accessed 14 April 2020].

[241] "Folic acid: vitamin that helps the body make healthy red blood cells", *nhs.uk*, 2019. [Online]. Available: https://www.nhs.uk/medicines/folic-acid/. [Accessed: 14- Apr- 2020].

[242] "Office of Dietary Supplements - Folate", *Ods.od.nih.gov*, 2020. [Online]. Available: https://ods.od.nih.gov/factsheets/Folate-HealthProfessional/. [Accessed: 30- Apr- 2020].

[243] "Folic Acid Safety, Interactions, and Effects on Other Outcomes", *Centers for Disease Control and Prevention*. [Online]. Available: https://www.cdc.gov/ncbddd/folicacid/faqs/faqs-safety.html. [Accessed: 11- May- 2020].

[244] "Table 1 Countries with mandatory folic acid fortification (as of...", *ResearchGate*, 2020. [Online]. Available: https://www.researchgate.net/figure/Countries-with-mandatory-folic-acid-fortification-as-of-October-2017-5_tbl1_322833299. [Accessed: 04- Jul- 2020].

[245] "Folic acid added to flour to prevent spinal conditions in babies", *GOV.UK*, 2021. [Online]. Available: https://www.gov.uk/government/news/folic-acid-added-to-flour-to-prevent-spinal-conditions-in-babies. [Accessed: 27- Sep- 2021].

[246] "Digitalis", *Ch.ic.ac.uk*. [Online]. Available: https://www.ch.ic.ac.uk/vchemlib/mim/bristol/digitalis/digitalis_text.htm#. [Accessed: 04- Jul- 2020].

[247] M. Sabater-Molina, E. Larqué, F. Torrella and S. Zamora, "Dietary fructooligosaccharides and potential benefits on health", *Journal of Physiology and Biochemistry*, vol. 65, no. 3, pp. 315-328, 2009. Available: https://link.springer.com/article/10.1007/BF03180584. [Accessed 16 April 2020].

[248] Y. Belkaid and T. Hand, "Role of the Microbiota in Immunity and Inflammation", *Cell*, vol. 157, no. 1, pp. 121-141, 2014. Available: https://www.ncbi.nlm.nih.gov/pmc/articles/PMC4056765/. [Accessed 16 April 2020].

[249] M. Sabater-Molina, E. Larqué, F. Torrella and S. Zamora, "Dietary fructooligosaccharides and potential benefits on health", *Journal of Physiology and Biochemistry*, vol. 65, no. 3, pp. 315-328, 2009. Available: https://pubmed.ncbi.nlm.nih.gov/20119826/. [Accessed 24 April 2020].

[250] J. Heo et al., "Gut microbiota Modulated by Probiotics and Garcinia cambogia Extract Correlate with Weight Gain and Adipocyte Sizes in High Fat-Fed Mice", *Scientific Reports*, vol. 6, no. 1, 2016. Available: https://www.nature.com/articles/srep33566/. [Accessed 17 April 2020].

[251] Q. Fan et al., "Garcinia cambogia extract removes calcium oxalate kidney stones in both genetic and non-genetic Drosophila models of nephrolithiasis", 2018. Available: https://www.biorxiv.org/content/10.1101/477570v1.abstract. [Accessed 17 April 2020].

[252] S. Heymsfield, D. Allison, J. Vasselli, A. Pietrobelli, D. Greenfield and C. Nunez, "Garcinia cambogia (Hydroxycitric Acid) as a Potential Antiobesity Agent", *JAMA*, vol. 280, no. 18, p. 1596, 1998. Available: https://jamanetwork.com/journals/jama/fullarticle/188147. [Accessed 3 June 2020].

[253] *Nccih.nih.gov*, 2016. [Online]. Available: https://www.nccih.nih.gov/health/garlic. [Accessed: 16- May- 2020].

[254] K. Srinivasan, "Ginger rhizomes (Zingiber officinale): A spice with multiple health beneficial potentials", *PharmaNutrition*, vol. 5, no. 1, pp. 18-28, 2017. Available: https://www.sciencedirect.com/science/article/pii/S2213434416300676. [Accessed 17 April 2020].

[255] H. Li et al., "Ginger for health care: An overview of systematic reviews", *Complementary Therapies in Medicine*, vol. 45, pp. 114-123, 2019. Available: https://www.sciencedirect.com/science/article/abs/pii/S0965229919303504. [Accessed 17 April 2020].

[256] *Nccih.nih.gov*, 2016. [Online]. Available: https://www.nccih.nih.gov/health/ginger. [Accessed: 16- May- 2020].

[257] C. Wang, S. Anderson, W. Du, T. He and C. Yuan, "Red ginseng and cancer treatment", *Sciencedirect.com*, 2016. [Online]. Available: https://www.sciencedirect.com/science/article/pii/S1875536416300048. [Accessed: 17- April- 2020].

[258] *Nccih.nih.gov*, 2016. [Online]. Available: https://www.nccih.nih.gov/health/asian-ginseng. [Accessed: 26- May- 2020].

[259] F. Au-Yeung, E. Jovanovski, A. Jenkins, A. Zurbau, H. Ho and V. Vuksan, "The effects of gelled konjac glucomannan fibre on appetite and energy intake in healthy individuals: a randomised cross-over trial", *British Journal of Nutrition*, vol. 119, no. 1, pp. 109-116, 2017. Available: https://doi.org/10.1017/S0007114517003233. [Accessed 16 April 2020].

[260] R. Tester and F. Al-Ghazzewi, "Glucomannans and nutrition", *Food Hydrocolloids*, vol. 68, pp. 246-254, 2017. Available: https://www.sciencedirect.com/science/article/pii/S0268005X16302144. [Accessed 16 April 2020].

[261] "The NIH Glucosamine/Chondroitin Arthritis Intervention Trial (GAIT)", *Journal of Pain & Palliative Care Pharmacotherapy*, vol. 22, no. 1, pp. 39-43, 2008. Available: https://pubmed.ncbi.nlm.nih.gov/19062354/. [Accessed 17 April 2020].

[262] T. Ogata et al., "Effects of glucosamine in patients with osteoarthritis of the knee: a systematic review and meta-analysis", *Clinical Rheumatology*, vol. 37, no. 9, pp. 2479-2487, 2018. Available: https://pubmed.ncbi.nlm.nih.gov/29713967/. [Accessed 16 May 2020].]

[263] O. Bruyere et al., "Total joint replacement after glucosamine sulphate treatment in knee osteoarthritis: results of a mean 8-year observation of patients from two previous 3-year, randomised, placebo-controlled trials", *Osteoarthritis and Cartilage*, vol. 16, no. 2, pp. 254-260, 2008. Available: https://pubmed.ncbi.nlm.nih.gov/17681803/. [Accessed 16 May 2020].

[264] M. Melzig, "Goldenrod – a classical exponent in the urological phytotherapy", *Wiener Medizinische Wochenschrift*, vol. 154, no. 21-22, pp. 523-527, 2004. Available: https://pubmed.ncbi.nlm.nih.gov/15638071/. [Accessed 4 June 2020].

[265] *Nccih.nih.gov*, 2016. [Online]. Available: https://www.nccih.nih.gov/health/goldenseal. [Accessed: 23- May- 2020].

[266] "Gotu Kola Uses, Benefits & Dosage - Drugs.com Herbal Database", *Drugs.com*, 2020. [Online]. Available: https://www.drugs.com/npp/gotu-kola.html. [Accessed: 17- Apr- 2020].

[267] V. Kedage, J. Tilak, G. Dixit, T. Devasagayam and M. Mhatre, "A Study of Antioxidant Properties of Some Varieties of Grapes (Vitis viniferaL.)", *Critical Reviews in Food Science and Nutrition*, vol. 47, no. 2, pp. 175-185, 2007. Available: https://pubmed.ncbi.nlm.nih.gov/17364701/. [Accessed 14 April 2020].

[268] H. Zhang et al., "The impact of grape seed extract treatment on blood pressure changes", *Medicine*, vol. 95, no. 33, p. e4247, 2016. Available: https://www.ncbi.nlm.nih.gov/pmc/articles/PMC5370781/. [Accessed 18 April 2020].

[269] "Grape: MedlinePlus Supplements", *Medlineplus.gov*, 2020. [Online]. Available: https://medlineplus.gov/druginfo/natural/472.html. [Accessed: 16- May- 2020].

[270] Y. Sun, C. Xiu, W. Liu, Y. Tao, J. Wang and Y. Qu, "Grape seed proanthocyanidin extract protects the retina against early diabetic injury by activating the Nrf2 pathway", *Experimental and Therapeutic Medicine*, vol. 11, no. 4, pp. 1253-1258, 2016. Available: http://10.3892/etm.2016.3033. [Accessed 16 May 2020].

[271] H. Feringa, D. Laskey, J. Dickson and C. Coleman, "The Effect of Grape Seed Extract on Cardiovascular Risk Markers: A Meta-Analysis of Randomized Controlled Trials", *Journal of the American Dietetic Association*, vol. 111, no. 8, pp. 1173-1181, 2011. Available: https://pubmed.ncbi.nlm.nih.gov/21802563/. [Accessed 16 May 2020].

[272] *Nccih.nih.gov*, 2020. [Online]. Available: https://www.nccih.nih.gov/health/grape-seed-extract. [Accessed: 16- May- 2020].

[273] S. Carrington, H. Fraser, J. Gilmore and G. Forde, *A-Z of Barbados heritage*. Oxford: Macmillan Caribbean, 2003, pp. pp. 90-91.

[274] H. Silver, M. Dietrich and K. Niswender, "Effects of grapefruit, grapefruit juice and water preloads on energy balance, weight loss, body composition, and cardiometabolic risk in free-living obese adults", *Nutrition & Metabolism*, vol. 8, no. 1, p. 8, 2011. Available: https://www.ncbi.nlm.nih.gov/pmc/articles/PMC3039556/. [Accessed 17 May 2020].

[275] K. Fujioka, F. Greenway, J. Sheard and Y. Ying, "The Effects of Grapefruit on Weight and Insulin Resistance: Relationship to the Metabolic Syndrome", *Journal of Medicinal Food*, vol. 9, no.

1, pp. 49-54, 2006. Available: https://pubmed.ncbi.nlm.nih.gov/16579728/. [Accessed 17 May 2020].

[276] "Brief History of Japanese Green Tea: A Cup Full of History and Mystery", *Japanese Green Tea www.JapaneseGreenTea.org*, 2020. [Online]. Available: https://www.japanesegreenteain.com/blogs/green-tea-and-health/brief-history-of-japanese-green-tea-a-cup-full-of-history-and-mystery#. [Accessed: 05- Jul- 2020].

[277] M. Barocio et al., "P148 The Administration of Green Tea Extract Improves Hemodynamic Parameters, Arterial Stiffness and Renal Function in Patients with Diabetic Nephropathy", *Artery Research*, vol. 25, no. 1, p. S185, 2020. Available: https://www.atlantis-press.com/journals/artres/125934605. [Accessed 24 May 2020].

[278] J. Hu, D. Webster, J. Cao and A. Shao, "The safety of green tea and green tea extract consumption in adults – Results of a systematic review", *Regulatory Toxicology and Pharmacology*, vol. 95, pp. 412-433, 2018. Available: https://www.sciencedirect.com/science/article/pii/S0273230018300928. [Accessed 17 April 2020].

[279] I. Chen, C. Liu, J. Chiu and C. Hsu, "Therapeutic effect of high-dose green tea extract on weight reduction: A randomized, double-blind, placebo-controlled clinical trial", *Clinical Nutrition*, vol. 35, no. 3, pp. 592-599, 2016. Available: https://www.clinicalnutritionjournal.com/article/S0261-5614(15)00134-X/fulltext. [Accessed 17 April 2020].

[280] S. Henning, et al, "Combination of Quercetin and Green Tea Extract Increased Plasma Epicatechingallate and Decreased Urine Epigallocatechin and Epicatechin Concentrations | The FASEB Journal", *Fasebj.org*, 2017. [Online]. Available: https://www.fasebj.org/doi/abs/10.1096/fasebj.31.1_supplement.148.8. [Accessed: 17- Apr- 2020].

[281] *Nccih.nih.gov*, 2020. [Online]. Available: https://www.nccih.nih.gov/health/green-tea. [Accessed: 24- May- 2020].

[282] "Definition of GUARANI", *Merriam-webster.com*, 2020. [Online]. Available: https://www.merriam-webster.com/dictionary/guarani. [Accessed: 17- May- 2020].

[283] N. Lima et al., "Modulatory Effects of Guarana (Paullinia cupana) on Adipogenesis", *Nutrients*, vol. 9, no. 6, p. 635, 2017. Available: https://www.mdpi.com/2072-6643/9/6/635. [Accessed 13 Aug 2021].

[284] Lima NDS, Teixeira L, Gambero A, and Ribeiro ML. "Guarana (Paullinia cupana) Stimulates Mitochondrial Biogenesis in Mice Fed High-Fat Diet", *Nutrients*, vol. 10, no. 2, p. 165, 2018. Available: https://www.mdpi.com/2072-6643/10/2/165. [Accessed 24 May 2020].

[285] "Definition and meaning of Bonsai - Bonsai Empire", *Bonsaiempire.com*. [Online]. Available: https://www.bonsaiempire.com/origin/what-is-bonsai. [Accessed: 04- Jun- 2020].

[286] A. Furey, M. Tassell, R. Kingston, D. Gilroy and M. Lehane, "Hawthorn (Crataegus spp.) in the treatment of cardiovascular disease", *Pharmacognosy Reviews*, vol. 4, no. 7, p. 32, 2010. Available: https://www.ncbi.nlm.nih.gov/pmc/articles/PMC3249900/. [Accessed 4 June 2020].

[287] *Nccih.nih.gov*, 2016. [Online]. Available: https://www.nccih.nih.gov/health/hawthorn.

[Accessed: 04- Jun- 2020].

[288] C. Serban, A. Sahebkar, S. Ursoniu, F. Andrica and M. Banach, "Effect of sour tea (Hibiscus sabdariffa L.) on arterial hypertension", *Journal of Hypertension*, vol. 33, no. 6, pp. 1119-1127, 2015. Available: https://pubmed.ncbi.nlm.nih.gov/25875025/. [Accessed 4 June 2020].

[289] A. Zbuchea, "Up-to-date use of honey for burns treatment", *PubMed Central (PMC)*, 2014. [Online]. Available: https://www.ncbi.nlm.nih.gov/pmc/articles/PMC4158441 [Accessed: 17- May- 2020].

[290] O. Oduwole, M. Meremikwu, A. Oyo-Ita and E. Udoh, "Honey for acute cough in children", *Cochrane Database of Systematic Reviews*, 2014. Available: https://pubmed.ncbi.nlm.nih.gov/25536086/. [Accessed 17 May 2020].

[291] "Honey: MedlinePlus Supplements", *Medlineplus.gov*, 2019. [Online]. Available: https://medlineplus.gov/druginfo/natural/738.html. [Accessed: 17- May- 2020].

[292] A. Oryan, E. Alemzadeh and A. Moshiri, "Biological properties and therapeutic activities of honey in wound healing: A narrative review and meta-analysis", *Journal of Tissue Viability*, vol. 25, no. 2, pp. 98-118, 2016. Available: https://pubmed.ncbi.nlm.nih.gov/26852154/. [Accessed 17 May 2020].

[293] *Mentalitch.com*. [Online]. Available: https://mentalitch.com/the-history-of-beer-in-china/. [Accessed: 05- Jun- 2020].

[294] I. Kyrou et al., "Effects of a hops (Humulus lupulus L.) dry extract supplement on self-reported depression, anxiety and stress levels in apparently healthy young adults: a randomized, placebo-controlled, double-blind, crossover pilot study", *HORMONES*, 2017. Available: https://pubmed.ncbi.nlm.nih.gov/28742505/. [Accessed 18 April 2020].

[295] E. Pritchard, "Fact File: The horse chestnut tree", *Country Living*, 2016. [Online]. Available: https://www.countryliving.com/uk/homes-interiors/gardens/a657/fact-file-horse-chestnut-tree/. [Accessed: 05- Jun- 2020].

[296] M. Pittler and E. Ernst, "Horse chestnut seed extract for chronic venous insufficiency", *The Cochrane Database of Systematic Reviews*, 2001. Available: https://pubmed.ncbi.nlm.nih.gov/23152216/. [Accessed 18 May 2020].

[297] *Nccih.nih.gov*, 2016. [Online]. Available: https://www.nccih.nih.gov/health/horse-chestnut. [Accessed: 18- May- 2020].

[298] D. Carneiro et al., "Randomized, Double-Blind Clinical Trial to Assess the Acute Diuretic Effect of Equisetum arvense (Field Horsetail) in Healthy Volunteers", *Evidence-Based Complementary and Alternative Medicine*, vol. 2014, pp. 1-8, 2014. Available: https://www.ncbi.nlm.nih.gov/pmc/articles/PMC3960516/. [Accessed 18 April 2020].

[299] M. Phillips et al., "Differentiating factors of intra-articular injectables have a meaningful impact on knee osteoarthritis outcomes: a network meta-analysis", *Knee Surgery, Sports Traumatology, Arthroscopy*, 2020. Available: https://link.springer.com/article/10.1007/s00167-019-05763-1. [Accessed: 18- Sept- 2021].

[300] "Vitamins and minerals - Iodine", *nhs.uk*, 2017. [Online]. Available: https://www.nhs.uk/conditions/vitamins-and-minerals/iodine/. [Accessed: 18- Apr- 2020].

[301] "Office of Dietary Supplements - Iodine", *Ods.od.nih.gov*, 2020. [Online]. Available: https://ods.od.nih.gov/factsheets/Iodine-HealthProfessional/. [Accessed: 30- Apr- 2020].

[302] "Scientific Opinion on the substantiation of a health claim related to "native chicory inulin"", *Efsa.onlinelibrary.wiley.com*, 2015. [Online]. Available: https://efsa.onlinelibrary.wiley.com/doi/epdf/10.2903/j.efsa.2015.3951. [Accessed: 18- Apr- 2020].

[303] R. Hutkins et al., "Prebiotics: why definitions matter", *Current Opinion in Biotechnology*, vol. 37, pp. 1-7, 2016. Available: https://www.ncbi.nlm.nih.gov/pmc/articles/PMC4744122/. [Accessed 1 May 2020].

[304] N. Abbaspour, R. Hurrell and R. Kelishadi, "Review on iron and its importance for human health", *PubMed Central (PMC)*, 2014. [Online]. Available: https://www.ncbi.nlm.nih.gov/pmc/articles/PMC3999603/. [Accessed: 27- Apr- 2020].

[305] F. Pizarro et al., "The effect of proteins from animal source foods on heme iron bioavailability in humans", *Food Chemistry*, vol. 196, pp. 733-738, 2016. Available: https://www.sciencedirect.com/science/article/abs/pii/S0308814615300121. [Accessed 27 April 2020].

[306] "Office of Dietary Supplements - Iron", *Ods.od.nih.gov*, 2020. [Online]. Available: https://ods.od.nih.gov/factsheets/Iron-HealthProfessional/. [Accessed: 05- Jun- 2020].

[307] "Final Report on the Safety Assessment of Juniperus Communis Extract, Juniperus Oxycedrus Extract, Juniperus Oxycedrus Tar, Juniperus Phoenicea Extract, and Juniperus Virginiana Extract", *International Journal of Toxicology*, vol. 20, no. 2, pp. 41-56, 2001. Available: https://pubmed.ncbi.nlm.nih.gov/11558640/. [Accessed 5 June 2020].

[308] "Juniper: Health Benefits, Uses, Side Effects, Dosage & Interactions", *RxList*. [Online]. Available: https://www.rxlist.com/juniper/supplements.htm. [Accessed: 05- Jun- 2020].

[309] "Office of Dietary Supplements - Vitamin K", *Ods.od.nih.gov*, 2020. [Online]. Available: https://ods.od.nih.gov/factsheets/vitaminK-HealthProfessional/. [Accessed: 30- Apr- 2020].

[310] J. Stenflo, P. Fernlund, W. Egan and P. Roepstorff, "Vitamin K Dependent Modifications of Glutamic Acid Residues in Prothrombin", *Proceedings of the National Academy of Sciences*, vol. 71, no. 7, pp. 2730-2733, 1974. Available: https://pubmed.ncbi.nlm.nih.gov/4528109/. [Accessed 19 April 2020].

[311] S. Magnusson, L. Sottrup-jensen and T. Petersen, "Primary structure of the vitamin K-dependent part of prothrombin", *FEBS Letters*, vol. 44, no. 2, pp. 189-193, 1974. Available: https://pubmed.ncbi.nlm.nih.gov/4472513/. [Accessed 19 April 2020].

[312] G. Nelsestuen, T. Zytkovicz and J. Howard, "The Mode of Action of Vitamin K. Identification of Gamma-Carboxyglutamic Acid as a Component of Prothrombin", *PubMed*, 1974. [Online]. Available: https://pubmed.ncbi.nlm.nih.gov/4214105/. [Accessed: 19- Apr- 2020].

[313] M. Shearer and P. Newman, "Metabolism and Cell Biology of Vitamin K", *PubMed*, 2008.

[Online]. Available: https://pubmed.ncbi.nlm.nih.gov/18841274/?dopt=Abstract [Accessed: 30- Apr- 2020].

[314] 2017. [Online]. Available: https://www.nhs.uk/conditions/vitamins-and-minerals/vitamin-k/. [Accessed: 12- Apr- 2021].

[315] "Vitamin K", *Ncbi.nlm.nih.gov*, 2001. [Online]. Available: https://www.ncbi.nlm.nih.gov/books/NBK222299/. [Accessed: 30- Apr- 2020].

[316] *Nccih.nih.gov*, 2016. [Online]. Available: https://www.nccih.nih.gov/health/kava. [Accessed: 15- May- 2020].

[317] T. Wernberg, K. Krumhansl, K. Filbee-Dexter and M. Pedersen, "Status and Trends for the World's Kelp Forests", *World Seas: an Environmental Evaluation*, pp. 57-78, 2019. Available: https://www.sciencedirect.com/science/article/pii/B9780128050521000036. [Accessed: 8 July 2020].

[318] S. Bor et al., "Alginates: From the ocean to gastroesophageal reflux disease treatment", *The Turkish Journal of Gastroenterology*, vol. 30, no. -2, pp. 109-136, 2019. Available: https://www.ncbi.nlm.nih.gov/pmc/articles/PMC6836317/. [Accessed 18 April 2020].

[319] "Bad Bug Book", pp 254-255, *Fda.gov*, 2020. [Online]. Available: https://www.fda.gov/media/83271/download. [Accessed: 05- Jun- 2020].

[320] S. Wang, L. Chen, H. Yang, J. Gu, J. Wang and F. Ren, "Regular intake of white kidney beans extract (Phaseolus vulgaris L.) induces weight loss compared to placebo in obese human subjects", *Food Science & Nutrition*, vol. 8, no. 3, pp. 1315-1324, 2020. Available: https://onlinelibrary.wiley.com/doi/full/10.1002/fsn3.1299. [Accessed 18 April 2020].

[321] J. Backes and P. Howard, "Krill Oil for Cardiovascular Risk Prevention: Is it for Real?", *Hospital Pharmacy*, vol. 49, no. 10, pp. 907-912, 2014. Available: https://www.ncbi.nlm.nih.gov/pmc/articles/PMC4252213/. [Accessed 18 April 2020].

[322] "Scientific Opinion on the substantiation of health claims related to L-glutamine", *Efsa.onlinelibrary.wiley.com*, 2011. [Online]. Available: https://efsa.onlinelibrary.wiley.com/doi/epdf/10.2903/j.efsa.2011.2225. [Accessed: 19- Apr- 2020].

[323] D. Whitbread, "Top 10 Foods Highest in Tyrosine", *myfooddata*, 2020. [Online]. Available: https://www.myfooddata.com/articles/high-tyrosine-foods.php. [Accessed: 19- Apr- 2020].

[324] R. Martín, S. Miquel, J. Ulmer, N. Kechaou, P. Langella and L. Bermúdez-Humarán, "Role of commensal and probiotic bacteria in human health: a focus on inflammatory bowel disease", *Microbial Cell Factories*, vol. 12, no. 1, p. 71, 2013. Available: https://www.ncbi.nlm.nih.gov/pmc/articles/PMC3726476/. [Accessed 19 April 2020].

[325] Z. Wang, Y. Yang, A. Stefka, G. Sun and L. Peng, "Review article: fungal microbiota and digestive diseases", *Alimentary Pharmacology & Therapeutics*, vol. 39, no. 8, pp. 751-766, 2014. Available: https://pubmed.ncbi.nlm.nih.gov/24612332/. [Accessed 19 April 2020].

[326] N. Martins, I. Ferreira, L. Barros, S. Silva and M. Henriques, "Candidiasis: Predisposing

Factors, Prevention, Diagnosis and Alternative Treatment", *Mycopathologia*, vol. 177, no. 5-6, pp. 223-240, 2014. Available: https://pubmed.ncbi.nlm.nih.gov/24789109/. [Accessed 19 April 2020].

[327] "Lactobacillus: MedlinePlus Supplements", *Medlineplus.gov*, 2019. [Online]. Available: https://medlineplus.gov/druginfo/natural/790.html. [Accessed: 18- Apr- 2020].

[328] S. Vlaisavljević et al., "Alchemilla vulgaris agg. (Lady's mantle) from central Balkan: antioxidant, anticancer and enzyme inhibition properties", *RSC Advances*, vol. 9, no. 64, pp. 37474-37483, 2019. Available: https://pubs.rsc.org/en/content/articlelanding/2019/ra/c9ra08231j#!divAbstract. [Accessed 7 June 2020].

[329] "Definition of OLD-WORLD", *Merriam-webster.com*, 2020. [Online]. Available: https://www.merriam-webster.com/dictionary/old-world?show=2&t=1417643287. [Accessed: 01- May- 2020].

[330] "The History of Lavender", *Tumalolavender.com*. [Online]. Available: https://www.tumalolavender.com/article-history-of-lavender.htm. [Accessed: 25- May- 2020].

[331] "Lavender Uses, Benefits & Dosage - Drugs.com Herbal Database", *Drugs.com*, 2018. [Online]. Available: https://www.drugs.com/npp/lavender.html. [Accessed: 01- May- 2020].

[332] I. Hay, M. Jamieson and A. Ormerod, "Randomized Trial of Aromatherapy", Archives of Dermatology, vol. 134, no. 11, 1998. Available: https://jamanetwork.com/journals/jamadermatology/fullarticle/189618. [Accessed 25 May 2020].

[333] D. Morris, "Flax – A Health and Nutrition Primer", *Flax Council Of Canada*, 2007. [Online]. Available: https://flaxcouncil.ca/resources/nutrition/technical-nutrition-information/flax-a-health-and-nutrition-primer/. [Accessed: 19- Apr- 2020].

[334] F. Størmer, R. Reistad and J. Alexander, "Glycyrrhizic acid in liquorice—Evaluation of health hazard", *Food and Chemical Toxicology*, vol. 31, no. 4, pp. 303-312, 1993. Available: https://pubmed.ncbi.nlm.nih.gov/8386690/. [Accessed 19 April 2020].

[335] C. Meilahti, "A new study confirms: pregnant women should avoid liquorice | University of Helsinki", *University of Helsinki*, 2017. [Online]. Available: https://www.helsinki.fi/en/news/health/a-new-study-confirms-pregnant-women-should-avoid-liquorice. [Accessed: 18- May- 2020].

[336] V. Liaugaudaite, N. Mickuviene, N. Raskauskiene, R. Naginiene and L. Sher, "Lithium levels in the public drinking water supply and risk of suicide: A pilot study", *Journal of Trace Elements in Medicine and Biology*, vol. 43, pp. 197-201, 2017. Available: https://www.sciencedirect.com/science/article/pii/S0946672X16302887. [Accessed 27 April 2020].

[337] L. Kessing et al., "Association of Lithium in Drinking Water with the Incidence of Dementia", *JAMA Psychiatry*, vol. 74, no. 10, p. 1005, 2017. Available: https://jamanetwork.com/journals/jamapsychiatry/fullarticle/2649277. [Accessed 27 April 2020].

[338] G. Schrauzer, "Lithium: Occurrence, Dietary Intakes, Nutritional Essentiality", *Journal of the American College of Nutrition*, vol. 21, no. 1, pp. 14-21, 2002. Available: https://

pubmed.ncbi.nlm.nih.gov/11838882/. [Accessed 27 April 2020].

[339] A. Naeem, M. Aslam, Saifullah and K. Mühling, "Lithium: Perspectives of nutritional beneficence, dietary intake, biogeochemistry, and biofortification of vegetables and mushrooms", Science of The Total Environment, vol. 798, p. 149249, 2021. Available: https://doi.org/10.1016/j.scitotenv.2021.149249. [Accessed 3 January 2022].

[340] V. Preedy, Essential oils in food preservation, flavor and safety. Academic Press, 2015, p. 540.

[341] U. Złotek, U. Szymanowska, Ł. Pecio, S. Kozachok and A. Jakubczyk, "Antioxidative and Potentially Anti-inflammatory Activity of Phenolics from Lovage Leaves Levisticum officinale Koch Elicited with Jasmonic Acid and Yeast Extract", *Molecules*, vol. 24, no. 7, p. 1441, 2019. Available: https://www.ncbi.nlm.nih.gov/pmc/articles/PMC6480578/. [Accessed 3 January 2022].

[342] D. GRAY and L. FOWDEN, "α-(Methylenecyclopropyl)glycine from Litchi seeds", Biochemical Journal, vol. 82, no. 3, pp. 385-389, 1962. Available: https://www.ncbi.nlm.nih.gov/pmc/articles/PMC1243468/. [Accessed 7 June 2020].

[343] M. Lee, H. Lee, S. You and K. Ha, "The use of maca (Lepidium meyenii) to improve semen quality: A systematic review", *Maturitas*, vol. 92, pp. 64-69, 2016. Available: https://pubmed.ncbi.nlm.nih.gov/27621241/. [Accessed 20 April 2020].

[344] M. Tam, S. Gómez, M. González-Gross and A. Marcos, "Possible roles of magnesium on the immune system", *European Journal of Clinical Nutrition*, vol. 57, no. 10, pp. 1193-1197, 2003. Available: https://www.nature.com/articles/1601689. [Accessed 27 April 2020].

[345] 2017. [Online]. Available: https://www.nhs.uk/conditions/vitamins-and-minerals/others/. [Accessed: 27- Apr- 2020].

[346] "Office of Dietary Supplements - Magnesium", *Ods.od.nih.gov*, 2020. [Online]. Available: https://ods.od.nih.gov/factsheets/Magnesium-HealthProfessional/. [Accessed: 01- May- 2020].

[347] A. Holley, V. Bakthavatchalu, J. Velez-Roman and D. St. Clair, "Manganese Superoxide Dismutase: Guardian of the Powerhouse", 2021. https://www.ncbi.nlm.nih.gov/pmc/articles/PMC3211030/ Accessed: [08- Oct- 2021].

[348] C. Godsey, D. Horowitz and R. Sather, "Manganese - Health Encyclopedia - University of Rochester Medical Center", *Urmc.rochester.edu*, 2020. [Online]. Available: https://www.urmc.rochester.edu/encyclopedia/content.aspx?contenttypeid=19&contentid=Manganese. [Accessed: 03- Jan- 2022].

[349] "Office of Dietary Supplements - Manganese", *Ods.od.nih.gov*, 2020. [Online]. Available: https://ods.od.nih.gov/factsheets/Manganese-HealthProfessional/. [Accessed: 01- May- 2020].

[350] N. Ortiz, "Saccharomyces Boulardii: A Yeast You Don't Want to Live Without! - Desert Health®", *Deserthealthnews.com*. [Online]. Available: https://deserthealthnews.com/stories/saccharomyces-boulardii-a-yeast-you-dont-want-to-live-without/. [Accessed: 07- Jun- 2020].

[351] J. Stern, J. Peerson, A. Mishra, V. Mathukumalli and P. Konda, "Efficacy and Tolerability

of an Herbal Formulation for Weight Management", *Journal of Medicinal Food*, vol. 16, no. 6, pp. 529-537, 2013. Available: https://www.ncbi.nlm.nih.gov/pmc/articles/PMC3684102/. [Accessed 18 May 2020].

[352] M. Raman and K. Gopakumar, *Ecronicon.com*, 2018. [Online]. Available: https://www.ecronicon.com/ecnu/pdf/ECNU-13-00529.pdf. [Accessed: 20- Apr- 2020].

[353] S. Boitsov, B. Grøsvik, G. Nesje, K. Malde and J. Klungsøyr, "Levels and temporal trends of persistent organic pollutants (POPs) in Atlantic cod (Gadus morhua) and haddock (Melanogrammus aeglefinus) from the southern Barents Sea", *Environmental Research*, vol. 172, pp. 89-97, 2019. Available: https://pubmed.ncbi.nlm.nih.gov/30782539/. [Accessed 5 May 2021].

[354] P. Rohdewald, "Review on Sustained Relief of Osteoarthritis Symptoms with a Proprietary Extract from Pine Bark, Pycnogenol", *Journal of Medicinal Food*, vol. 21, no. 1, pp. 1-4, 2018. Available: https://www.liebertpub.com/doi/full/10.1089/jmf.2017.0015. [Accessed 24 April 2020].

[355] A. Hadi, M. Pourmasoumi, H. Mohammadi, A. Javaheri and M. Rouhani, "The impact of pycnogenol supplementation on plasma lipids in humans: A systematic review and meta-analysis of clinical trials", *Phytotherapy Research*, vol. 33, no. 2, pp. 276-287, 2018. Available: https://onlinelibrary.wiley.com/doi/abs/10.1002/ptr.6234. [Accessed 4 January 2022].

[356] "Maritime Pine: MedlinePlus Supplements", *Medlineplus.gov*, 2019. [Online]. Available: https://medlineplus.gov/druginfo/natural/1019.html. [Accessed: 18- May- 2020].

[357] O. Said, S. Fulder, K. Khalil, H. Azaizeh, E. Kassis and B. Saad, "Maintaining a Physiological Blood Glucose Level with 'Glucolevel', a Combination of Four Anti-Diabetes Plants Used in the Traditional Arab Herbal Medicine", *Evidence-Based Complementary and Alternative Medicine*, vol. 5, no. 4, pp. 421-428, 2008. Available: http://downloads.hindawi.com/journals/ecam/2008/720130.pdf. [Accessed 10 April 2020].

[358] *Nccih.nih.gov*, 2016. [Online]. Available: https://www.nccih.nih.gov/health/milkthistle. [Accessed: 18- May- 2020].

[359] S. Foong, M. Tan, L. Marasco, J. Ho and W. Foong, "Oral galactagogues for increasing breast-milk production in mothers of non-hospitalised term infants", *Cochrane Database of Systematic Reviews*, 2015. Available: https://www.cochranelibrary.com/cdsr/doi/10.1002/14651858.CD011505/full. [Accessed 18 May 2020].

[360] J. Novotny and C. Peterson, "Molybdenum", Advances in Nutrition, vol. 9, no. 3, pp. 272-273, 2018. Available: https://academic.oup.com/advances/article/9/3/272/4996100. [Accessed 28 April 2020].

[361] C. Kisker, H. Schindelin, D. Baas, J. Rétey, R. Meckenstock and P. Kroneck, "A structural comparison of molybdenum cofactor-containing enzymes", *FEMS Microbiology Reviews*, vol. 22, no. 5, pp. 503-521, 1998. Available: https://pubmed.ncbi.nlm.nih.gov/9990727/. [Accessed 28 April 2020].

[362] [3]C. Yang, "Research on Esophageal Cancer in China: A Review", *PubMed*, 2020. [On-

line]. Available: https://pubmed.ncbi.nlm.nih.gov/6992989/. [Accessed: 28- Apr- 2020].

[363] "Office of Dietary Supplements - Molybdenum", *Ods.od.nih.gov*, 2020. [Online]. Available: https://ods.od.nih.gov/factsheets/Molybdenum-HealthProfessional/. [Accessed: 01- May- 2020].

[364] P. Morgan, M. Barton and J. Bowtell, "Montmorency cherry supplementation improves 15-km cycling time-trial performance", *European Journal of Applied Physiology*, vol. 119, no. 3, pp. 675-684, 2019. Available: https://link.springer.com/article/10.1007/s00421-018-04058-6. [Accessed 4 January 2022].

[365] Z. Aboo Bakkar et al., "Montmorency cherry supplementation attenuates vascular dysfunction induced by prolonged forearm occlusion in overweight, middle-aged men", *Journal of Applied Physiology*, vol. 126, no. 1, pp. 246-254, 2019. Available: https://journals.physiology.org/doi/full/10.1152/japplphysiol.00804.2018. [Accessed 20 April 2020].

[366] D. Kelley, Y. Adkins and K. Laugero, "A Review of the Health Benefits of Cherries", *Nutrients*, vol. 10, no. 3, p. 368, 2018. Available: https://www.ncbi.nlm.nih.gov/pmc/articles/PMC5872786/. [Accessed 7 June 2020].

[367] "Horseradish-tree, leafy tips, cooked, boiled, drained, without salt Nutrition Facts & Calories", *Nutritiondata.self.com*, 2020. [Online]. Available: https://nutritiondata.self.com/facts/vegetables-and-vegetable-products/2453/2. [Accessed: 20- Apr- 2020].

[368] G. Michon, *Numericana.com*, 2020. [Online]. Available: http://www.numericana.com/answer/culture.htm. [Accessed: 07- Jun- 2020].

[369] L. Kim, L. Axelrod, P. Howard, N. Buratovich and R. Waters, "Efficacy of methylsulfonylmethane (MSM) in osteoarthritis pain of the knee: a pilot clinical trial", *Osteoarthritis and Cartilage*, vol. 14, no. 3, pp. 286-294, 2006. Available: https://pubmed.ncbi.nlm.nih.gov/16309928/. [Accessed 20 April 2020].

[370] P. Usha and M. Naidu, "Randomised, Double-Blind, Parallel, Placebo-Controlled Study of Oral Glucosamine, Methylsulfonylmethane and their Combination in Osteoarthritis", *Clinical Drug Investigation*, vol. 24, no. 6, pp. 353-363, 2004. Available: https://pubmed.ncbi.nlm.nih.gov/17516722/. [Accessed 20 April 2020].

[371] A. Lubis, C. Siagian, E. Wonggokusuma, A. Marsetyo and B. Setyohadi, "Comparison of Glucosamine-Chondroitin Sulfate With and Without Methylsulfonylmethane in Grade I-II Knee Osteoarthritis: A Double Blind Randomized Controlled Trial", *PubMed*, 2017. [Online]. Available: https://pubmed.ncbi.nlm.nih.gov/28790224/. [Accessed: 08- Jun- 2020].

[372] M. Butawan, R. Benjamin and R. Bloomer, "Methylsulfonylmethane: Applications and Safety of a Novel Dietary Supplement", *Nutrients*, vol. 9, no. 3, p. 290, 2017. Available: https://www.ncbi.nlm.nih.gov/pmc/articles/PMC5372953/. [Accessed 28 April 2020].

[373] *Bio.utexas.edu*. [Online]. Available: http://www.bio.utexas.edu/courses/evolution/crowneuks1.pdf. [Accessed: 20- May- 2021].

[374] S. Baldauf and J. Palmer, "Animals and fungi are each other's closest relatives: congru-

ent evidence from multiple proteins.", 2022. [Online]. Available: https://pubmed.ncbi.nlm.nih.gov/8265589/. [Accessed: 04- Jan- 2022].

[375] R. Jäpelt and J. Jakobsen, "Vitamin D in plants: a review of occurrence, analysis, and biosynthesis", *Frontiers in Plant Science*, vol. 4, 2013. Available: https://www.ncbi.nlm.nih.gov/pmc/articles/PMC3651966/. [Accessed 20 April 2020].

[376] L. M and P. G, "Penicillin's Discovery and Antibiotic Resistance: Lessons for the Future?", *PubMed*, 2020. [Online]. Available: https://www.ncbi.nlm.nih.gov/pubmed/28356901. [Accessed: 04- Jan- 2022].

[377] "Alexander Fleming Discovery and Development of Penicillin - Landmark - American Chemical Society", *American Chemical Society*, 2020. [Online]. Available: https://www.acs.org/content/acs/en/education/whatischemistry/landmarks/flemingpenicillin.html. [Accessed: 04- Jan- 2022].

[378] T. Shonte and H. de Kock, "Descriptive sensory evaluation of cooked stinging nettle (Urtica dioica L.) leaves and leaf infusions: Effect of using fresh or oven-dried leaves", *South African Journal of Botany*, vol. 110, pp. 167-176, 2017. Available: https://www.sciencedirect.com/science/article/pii/S0254629916339448. [Accessed 21 April 2020].

[379] S. Vogl et al., "Ethnopharmacological in vitro studies on Austria's folk medicine—An unexplored lore in vitro anti-inflammatory activities of 71 Austrian traditional herbal drugs", *Journal of Ethnopharmacology*, vol. 149, no. 3, pp. 750-771, 2013. Available: https://pubmed.ncbi.nlm.nih.gov/23770053/. [Accessed 21 April 2020].

[380] "Nettle - Herbal Encyclopedia", *Healthmedicinet.com*. [Online]. Available: http://healthmedicinet.com/druginfo/natural/nettle/index.html. [Accessed: 08- Jun- 2020].

[381] D. Kregiel, E. Pawlikowska and H. Antolak, "Urtica spp.: Ordinary Plants with Extraordinary Properties", *Molecules*, vol. 23, no. 7, p. 1664, 2018. Available: https://www.ncbi.nlm.nih.gov/pmc/articles/PMC6100552/. [Accessed 21 April 2020].

[382] H. Akbari et al., "The Healing Effect of Nettle Extract on Second Degree Burn Wounds", *PubMed*, 2015. [Online]. Available: https://pubmed.ncbi.nlm.nih.gov/25606473/. [Accessed: 08- Jun- 2020].

[383] S. Klingelhoefer, B. Obertreis, S. Quast and B. Behnke, "Antirheumatic Effect of IDS 23, a Stinging Nettle Leaf Extract, on in Vitro Expression of T Helper Cytokines", *PubMed*, 1999. [Online]. Available: https://pubmed.ncbi.nlm.nih.gov/10606356/. [Accessed: 21- Apr- 2020].

[384] *Nccih.nih.gov*, 2016. [Online]. Available: https://www.nccih.nih.gov/health/noni. [Accessed: 20- May- 2020].

[385] "The Noni Website - Chemical Constituents of Noni", *Ctahr.hawaii.edu*, 2006. [Online]. Available: https://www.ctahr.hawaii.edu/noni/nutritional_analysis.asp. [Accessed: 20- May- 2020].

[386] P. Vossen, "Olive Oil: History, Production, and Characteristics of the World's Classic Oils", *HortScience*, vol. 42, no. 5, pp. 1093-1100, 2007. Available: https://journals.ashs.org/

hortsci/view/journals/hortsci/42/5/article-p1093.xml. [Accessed 8 June 2020].

[387] I. Therios, *Olives*. Cambridge, MA: CABI, 2009.

[388] "Showing report on Oils - Phenol-Explorer", *Phenol-explorer.eu*. [Online]. Available: http://phenol-explorer.eu/reports/45#olive. [Accessed: 22- Apr- 2020].

[389] C. Blesso, "Dietary Anthocyanins and Human Health", *Nutrients*, vol. 11, no. 9, p. 2107, 2019. Available: https://www.mdpi.com/2072-6643/11/9/2107. [Accessed 22 April 2020].

[390] W. Sun, B. Frost and J. Liu, "Oleuropein, unexpected benefits!", *Oncotarget*, vol. 8, no. 11, pp. 17409-17409, 2017. Available: https://www.ncbi.nlm.nih.gov/pmc/articles/PMC5392257/. [Accessed 04 January 2022].

[391] P. Lins, S. Marina Piccoli Pugine, A. Scatolini and M. de Melo, "In vitro antioxidant activity of olive leaf extract (Olea europaea L.) and its protective effect on oxidative damage in human erythrocytes", *Heliyon*, vol. 4, no. 9, p. e00805, 2018. Available: https://www.sciencedirect.com/science/article/pii/S2405844018318887. [Accessed 22 April 2020].

[392] G. H, "Can Adults Adequately Convert Alpha-Linolenic Acid (18:3n-3) to Eicosapentaenoic Acid (20:5n-3) and Docosahexaenoic Acid (22:6n-3)?", *PubMed*, 1998. [Online]. Available: https://pubmed.ncbi.nlm.nih.gov/9637947/. [Accessed: 01- May- 2020].

[393] K. Sheppard and C. Cheatham, "Omega-6/omega-3 fatty acid intake of children and older adults in the U.S.: dietary intake in comparison to current dietary recommendations and the Healthy Eating Index", *Lipids in Health and Disease*, vol. 17, no. 1, 2018. Available: https://www.ncbi.nlm.nih.gov/pmc/articles/PMC5845148/. [Accessed 1 May 2020].

[394] "Scientific Opinion on the Tolerable Upper Intake Level of eicosapentaenoic acid (EPA), docosahexaenoic acid (DHA) and docosapentaenoic acid (DPA)", *Efsa.onlinelibrary.wiley.com*, 2012. [Online]. Available: https://efsa.onlinelibrary.wiley.com/doi/epdf/10.2903/j.efsa.2012.2815. [Accessed: 11- May- 2020].

[395] "Essential Fatty Acids Intake Recommendations - NUTRI-FACTS", *Nutri-facts.org*, 2017. [Online]. Available: https://www.nutri-facts.org/en_US/nutrients/essential-fatty-acids/essential-fatty-acids/intake-recommendations.html. [Accessed: 01- May- 2020].

[396] Salami, "Oleic Acid - an overview | ScienceDirect Topics", *Sciencedirect.com*, 2016. [Online]. Available: https://www.sciencedirect.com/topics/food-science/oleic-acid. [Accessed: 01- May- 2020].

[397] "Oregano: MedlinePlus Supplements", *Medlineplus.gov*, 2019. [Online]. Available: https://medlineplus.gov/druginfo/natural/644.html. [Accessed: 22- Apr- 2020].

[398] H. Sakkas and C. Papadopoulou, "Antimicrobial Activity of Basil, Oregano, and Thyme Essential Oils", *Journal of Microbiology and Biotechnology*, vol. 27, no. 3, pp. 429-438, 2017. Available: http://www.jmb.or.kr/submission/Journal/027/JMB027-03-02_FDOC_1.pdf. [Accessed 22 April 2020].

[399] P. Kubatka et al., "Oregano demonstrates distinct tumour-suppressive effects in the breast carcinoma model", *European Journal of Nutrition*, vol. 56, no. 3, pp. 1303-1316, 2016.

Available: https://link.springer.com/article/10.1007/s00394-016-1181-5. [Accessed 22 April 2020].

[400] "Oregano: MedlinePlus Supplements", *Medlineplus.gov*, 2019. [Online]. Available: https://medlineplus.gov/druginfo/natural/644.html. [Accessed: 22- Apr- 2020].

[401] "Spices, parsley, dried Nutrition Facts & Calories", *Nutritiondata.self.com*. [Online]. Available: https://nutritiondata.self.com/facts/spices-and-herbs/199/2. [Accessed: 04- Jan- 2022].

[402] M. Farzaei, Z. Abbasabadi, M. Ardekani, R. Rahimi and F. Farzaei, "Parsley: a review of ethnopharmacology, phytochemistry and biological activities", *Journal of Traditional Chinese Medicine*, vol. 33, no. 6, pp. 815-826, 2013. Available: https://pubmed.ncbi.nlm.nih.gov/24660617/. [Accessed 9 June 2020].

[403] M. Barac et al., "Profile and Functional Properties of Seed Proteins from Six Pea (Pisum sativum) Genotypes", *International Journal of Molecular Sciences*, vol. 11, no. 12, pp. 4973-4990, 2010. Available: https://www.ncbi.nlm.nih.gov/pmc/articles/PMC3100834/. [Accessed 22 April 2020].

[404] *Motherearthnews.com*, 2008. [Online]. Available: https://www.motherearthnews.com/natural-health/herbal-remedies/pennyroyal-safety. [Accessed: 04- Jan- 2022].

[405] S. Hewlings and D. Kalman, "Curcumin: A Review of Its' Effects on Human Health", *Foods*, vol. 6, no. 10, p. 92, 2017. Available: https://www.ncbi.nlm.nih.gov/pmc/articles/PMC5664031/. [Accessed 23 April 2020].

[406] S. Butler, "Off the Spice Rack: The Story of Pepper", *HISTORY*, 2018. [Online]. Available: https://www.history.com/news/off-the-spice-rack-the-story-of-pepper. [Accessed: 09- Jun- 2020].

[407] Khanna R, MacDonald JK, Levesque BG. "Peppermint oil for the treatment of irritable bowel syndrome: a systematic review and meta-analysis." *J Clin Gastroenterol*. 2014;48(6):505-512. https://pubmed.ncbi.nlm.nih.gov/24100754/ [Accessed: 04- Jan- 2022]

[408] *Nccih.nih.gov*, 2016. [Online]. Available: https://www.nccih.nih.gov/health/peppermint-oil. [Accessed: 25- May- 2020].

[409] T. Takemoto et al., "Pfaffic acid, a novel nortriterpene from Pfaffia paniculata Kuntze", *Tetrahedron Letters*, vol. 24, no. 10, pp. 1057-1060, 1983. Available: https://www.sciencedirect.com/science/article/pii/S0040403900816032. [Accessed 10 June 2020].

[410] L. Taylor, "The Healing Power of Rainforest Herbs", *Rain-tree.com*, 2005. [Online]. Available: https://rain-tree.com/book2.htm. [Accessed: 10- Jun- 2020].

[411] C. Costa, A. Quaglio and L. Di Stasi, "Pfaffia paniculata (Brazilian ginseng) extract modulates Mapk and mucin pathways in intestinal inflammation", *Journal of Ethnopharmacology*, vol. 213, pp. 21-25, 2018. Available: https://www.sciencedirect.com/science/article/abs/pii/S0378874117320585. [Accessed 24 April 2020].

[412] "Nutrition's dynamic duos - Harvard Health", *Harvard Health*, 2009. [Online]. Avail-

able: https://www.health.harvard.edu/newsletter_article/Nutritions-dynamic-duos. [Accessed: 28- Apr- 2020].

[413] R. Bertram, M. Gram Pedersen, D. Luciani and A. Sherman, "A simplified model for mitochondrial ATP production", *Journal of Theoretical Biology*, vol. 243, no. 4, pp. 575-586, 2006. Available: https://pubmed.ncbi.nlm.nih.gov/16945388/. [Accessed 28 April 2020].

[414] "Office of Dietary Supplements - Phosphorus", *Ods.od.nih.gov*, 2019. [Online]. Available: https://ods.od.nih.gov/factsheets/Phosphorus-Consumer/. [Accessed: 28- Apr- 2020].

[415] "Office of Dietary Supplements - Phosphorus", *Ods.od.nih.gov*, 2020. [Online]. Available: https://ods.od.nih.gov/factsheets/Phosphorus-HealthProfessional/. [Accessed: 28- Apr- 2020].

[416] "Pomegranates, raw Nutrition Facts & Calories", *Nutritiondata.self.com*. [Online]. Available: https://nutritiondata.self.com/facts/fruits-and-fruit-juices/2038/2. [Accessed: 24- April- 2020].

[417] B. Singh, J. Singh, A. Kaur and N. Singh, "Phenolic compounds as beneficial phytochemicals in pomegranate (Punica granatum L.) peel: A review", Food Chemistry, vol. 261, pp. 75-86, 2018. Available: https://pubmed.ncbi.nlm.nih.gov/29739608/. [Accessed: 5- May- 2021].

[418] C. Kamau, *Etd.ohiolink.edu*, 2007. [Online]. Available: https://etd.ohiolink.edu/!etd.send_file?accession=bgsu1182707084&disposition=inline. [Accessed: 24- Apr- 2020].

[419] H. Zeweil, S. Elnagar, S. Zahran, M. Ahmed and Y. El-Gindy, "Pomegranate peel as a natural antioxidant boosts bucks' fertility under Egyptian summer conditions", World Rabbit Science, vol. 21, no. 1, 2013. Available: https://www.researchgate.net/publication/259532513_Pomegranate_peel_as_a_natural_antioxidant_boosts_bucks'_fertility_under_Egyptian_summer_conditions. [Accessed 24 April 2020].

[420] M. Nikseresht, "Effects of Pomegranate Seed Oil on the Fertilization Potency of Rat's Sperm", *JOURNAL OF CLINICAL AND DIAGNOSTIC RESEARCH*, 2015. Available: https://www.ncbi.nlm.nih.gov/pmc/articles/PMC4717727/. [Accessed 10 June 2020].

[421] M. Aviram and M. Rosenblat, "Pomegranate for Your Cardiovascular Health", *Rambam Maimonides Medical Journal*, vol. 4, no. 2, p. e0013, 2013. Available: https://www.ncbi.nlm.nih.gov/pmc/articles/PMC3678830/. [Accessed 10 June 2020].

[422] *Nccih.nih.gov*, 2016. [Online]. Available: https://www.nccih.nih.gov/health/pomegranate. [Accessed: 25- May- 2020].

[423] C. Meadway, S. George and R. Braithwaite, "Opiate concentrations following the ingestion of poppy seed products – evidence for `the poppy seed defence'", *Forensic Science International*, vol. 96, no. 1, pp. 29-38, 1998. Available: https://pubmed.ncbi.nlm.nih.gov/9800363/. [Accessed 28 April 2020].

[424] M. Brownstein, "A brief history of opiates, opioid peptides, and opioid receptors.", *Proceedings of the National Academy of Sciences*, vol. 90, no. 12, pp. 5391-5393, 1993. Available: https://www.ncbi.nlm.nih.gov/pmc/articles/PMC46725/. [Accessed 28 April 2020].

[425] "In Flanders Fields by John McCrae | Poetry Foundation", Poetry Foundation, 2022.

[Online]. Available: https://www.poetryfoundation.org/poems/47380/in-flanders-fields. [Accessed: 04- Jan- 2022].

[426] E. Ferrannini, A. Galvan, D. Santoro and A. Natali, "Potassium as a link between insulin and the renin-angiotensin-aldosterone system", *Journal of Hypertension*, vol. 10, no. 1, pp. S5-S10, 1992. Available: https://pubmed.ncbi.nlm.nih.gov/1619503/. [Accessed 24 April 2020].

[427] "Food Data Chart - Potassium", *Apjcn.nhri.org.tw*. [Online]. Available: http://apjcn.nhri.org.tw/server/info/books-phds/books/foodfacts/html/data/data5b.html. [Accessed: 24- Apr- 2020].

[428] "Potassium in diet: MedlinePlus Medical Encyclopedia", *Medlineplus.gov*, 2020. [Online]. Available: https://medlineplus.gov/ency/article/002413.htm. [Accessed: 28- Apr- 2020].

[429] "Office of Dietary Supplements - Potassium", *Ods.od.nih.gov*, 2020. [Online]. Available: https://ods.od.nih.gov/factsheets/Potassium-HealthProfessional/. [Accessed: 04- Dec- 2021].

[430] H. Holscher, "Dietary fiber and prebiotics and the gastrointestinal microbiota", *Gut Microbes*, vol. 8, no. 2, pp. 172-184, 2017. Available: https://www.ncbi.nlm.nih.gov/pmc/articles/PMC5390821/. [Accessed 24 April 2020].

[431] R. Hutkins et al., "Prebiotics: why definitions matter", *Current Opinion in Biotechnology*, vol. 37, pp. 1-7, 2016. Available: https://pubmed.ncbi.nlm.nih.gov/26431716/. [Accessed 7 May 2020].

[432] M. Mohajeri et al., "The role of the microbiome for human health: from basic science to clinical applications", *European Journal of Nutrition*, vol. 57, no. 1, pp. 1-14, 2018. Available: https://www.ncbi.nlm.nih.gov/pmc/articles/PMC5962619/. [Accessed 7 May 2020].

[433] D. Davani-Davari et al., "Prebiotics: Definition, Types, Sources, Mechanisms, and Clinical Applications", *Foods*, vol. 8, no. 3, p. 92, 2019. Available: https://www.ncbi.nlm.nih.gov/pmc/articles/PMC6463098/. [Accessed 7 May 2020].

[434] "List of Herbs in the NLM Herb Garden", *Nlm.nih.gov*, 2018. [Online]. Available: https://www.nlm.nih.gov/about/herbgarden/list.html. [Accessed: 28- Apr- 2020].

[435] J. König and R. Brummer, "Alteration of the intestinal microbiota as a cause of and a potential therapeutic option in irritable bowel syndrome", *Beneficial Microbes*, vol. 5, no. 3, pp. 247-261, 2014. Available: https://pubmed.ncbi.nlm.nih.gov/24583610/. [Accessed 7 May 2020].

[436] M. Ritchie and T. Romanuk, "A Meta-Analysis of Probiotic Efficacy for Gastrointestinal Diseases", *PLoS ONE*, vol. 7, no. 4, p. e34938, 2012. Available: https://www.ncbi.nlm.nih.gov/pmc/articles/PMC3329544/. [Accessed 12 June 2020].

[437] M. Kechagia et al., "Health Benefits of Probiotics: A Review", *ISRN Nutrition*, vol. 2013, pp. 1-7, 2013. Available: https://www.ncbi.nlm.nih.gov/pmc/articles/PMC4045285/. [Accessed 12 June 2020].

[438] M. Katzman and A. Logan, "Quo Vadis, Probiotics? Human Research Supports Further Study of Beneficial Microbes in Mental Health", *EBioMedicine*, vol. 24, pp. 14-15, 2017. Available: https://www.thelancet.com/article/S2352-3964(17)30372-9/fulltext. [Accessed 7 May 2020].

[439] 2018. [Online]. Available: https://fdc.nal.usda.gov/fdc-app.html#/food-details/168162/nutrients. [Accessed: 12- Jun- 2020].

[440] M. Stacewicz-Sapuntzakis, P. Bowen, E. Hussain, B. Damayanti-Wood and N. Farnsworth, "Chemical Composition and Potential Health Effects of Prunes: A Functional Food?", *Critical Reviews in Food Science and Nutrition*, vol. 41, no. 4, pp. 251-286, 2001. Available: https://www.tandfonline.com/doi/abs/10.1080/20014091091814. [Accessed 12 June 2020].

[441] K. Lambeau and J. McRorie, "Fiber supplements and clinically proven health benefits", *Journal of the American Association of Nurse Practitioners*, vol. 29, no. 4, pp. 216-223, 2017. Available: https://www.ncbi.nlm.nih.gov/pmc/articles/PMC5413815/. [Accessed 15 May 2020].

[442] "Tannin | biochemistry", *Encyclopedia Britannica*, 2020. [Online]. Available: https://www.britannica.com/science/tannin. [Accessed: 12- Jun- 2020].

[443] G. D'Andrea, "Quercetin: A flavonol with multifaceted therapeutic applications?", *Fitoterapia*, vol. 106, pp. 256-271, 2015. Available: https://pubmed.ncbi.nlm.nih.gov/26393898/. [Accessed 25 April 2020].

[444] B. Pickersgill, "Domestication of Plants in the Americas: Insights from Mendelian and Molecular Genetics", *Annals of Botany*, vol. 100, no. 5, pp. 925-940, 2007. Available: https://pubmed.ncbi.nlm.nih.gov/17766847/. [Accessed 25 April 2020].

[445] 2017. [Online]. Available: https://www.nhs.uk/conditions/vitamins-and-minerals/vitamin-c/. [Accessed: 25- Apr- 2020].

[446] B. Burton-Freeman, A. Sandhu and I. Edirisinghe, "Red Raspberries and Their Bioactive Polyphenols: Cardiometabolic and Neuronal Health Links", *Advances in Nutrition*, vol. 7, no. 1, pp. 44-65, 2016. Available: https://pubmed.ncbi.nlm.nih.gov/26773014/. [Accessed 25 April 2020].

[447] C. Bodinet and J. Freudenstein, "Influence of marketed herbal menopause preparations on MCF-7 cell proliferation", *Menopause*, vol. 11, no. 3, pp. 281-289, 2004. Available: https://pubmed.ncbi.nlm.nih.gov/15167307/. [Accessed 25 April 2020].

[448] 2019. [Online]. Available: https://fdc.nal.usda.gov/fdc-app.html#/food-details/168998/nutrients. [Accessed: 25- Apr- 2020].

[449] R. Christensen, E. Bartels, R. Altman, A. Astrup and H. Bliddal, "Does the hip powder of Rosa canina (rosehip) reduce pain in osteoarthritis patients? – a meta-analysis of randomized controlled trials", *Osteoarthritis and Cartilage*, vol. 16, no. 9, pp. 965-972, 2008. Available: https://pubmed.ncbi.nlm.nih.gov/18407528/. [Accessed 25 April 2020].

[450] S. Petiwala, A. Puthenveetil and J. Johnson, "Polyphenols from the Mediterranean herb rosemary (Rosmarinus officinalis) for prostate cancer", *Frontiers in Pharmacology*, vol. 4, 2013. Available: https://pubmed.ncbi.nlm.nih.gov/23531917/. [Accessed 25 April 2020].

[451] M. Ramadan and A. Al-Ghamdi, "Bioactive compounds and health-promoting properties of royal jelly: A review", *Journal of Functional Foods*, vol. 4, no. 1, pp. 39-52, 2012. Available: https://www.sciencedirect.com/science/article/pii/S1756464611001137. [Accessed 25 April 2020].

[452] 2020. [Online]. Available: https://fdc.nal.usda.gov/fdc-app.html#/food-details/786745/nutrients. [Accessed: 25- Apr- 2020].

[453] *Nccih.nih.gov*, 2016. [Online]. Available: https://www.nccih.nih.gov/health/sage. [Accessed: 26- Apr- 2020].

[454] A. Lopresti, "Salvia (Sage): A Review of its Potential Cognitive-Enhancing and Protective Effects", *Drugs in R&D*, vol. 17, no. 1, pp. 53-64, 2016. Available: https://www.ncbi.nlm.nih.gov/pmc/articles/PMC5318325/. [Accessed 26 April 2020].

[455] "Selenium", *Linus Pauling Institute*, 2020. [Online]. Available: https://lpi.oregonstate.edu/mic/minerals/selenium. [Accessed: 25- Apr- 2020].

[456] E. Zoidis, I. Seremelis, N. Kontopoulos and G. Danezis, "Selenium-Dependent Antioxidant Enzymes: Actions and Properties of Selenoproteins", *Antioxidants*, vol. 7, no. 5, p. 66, 2018. Available: https://www.ncbi.nlm.nih.gov/pmc/articles/PMC5981252/. [Accessed 14 June 2020].

[457] "Office of Dietary Supplements - Selenium", *Ods.od.nih.gov*, 2019. [Online]. Available: https://ods.od.nih.gov/factsheets/Selenium-Consumer/. [Accessed: 27- Apr- 2020].

[458] J. Geleijnse, F. Kok and D. Grobbee, "Impact of dietary and lifestyle factors on the prevalence of hypertension in Western populations", *The European Journal of Public Health*, vol. 14, no. 3, pp. 235-239, 2004. Available: https://pubmed.ncbi.nlm.nih.gov/15369026/. [Accessed 28 April 2020].

[459] "Learn About... Sorrel", *Urban Cultivator*. [Online]. Available: https://www.urbancultivator.net/learn-about-sorrell/. [Accessed: 14- Jun- 2020].

[460] "Calcium Oxalate Stones", *National Kidney Foundation*, 2020. [Online]. Available: https://www.kidney.org/atoz/content/calcium-oxalate-stone. [Accessed: 28- Apr- 2020].

[461] G. Lee, G. Crawford, L. Liu, Y. Sasaki and X. Chen, "Archaeological Soybean (Glycine max) in East Asia: Does Size Matter?", *PLoS ONE*, vol. 6, no. 11, p. e26720, 2011. Available: https://pubmed.ncbi.nlm.nih.gov/22073186/. [Accessed 27 April 2020].

[462] [2]J. Harland and T. Haffner, "Systematic review, meta-analysis and regression of randomised controlled trials reporting an association between an intake of circa 25g soya protein per day and blood cholesterol", *Atherosclerosis*, vol. 200, no. 1, pp. 13-27, 2008. Available: https://pubmed.ncbi.nlm.nih.gov/18534601/. [Accessed 27 April 2020].

[463] M. Baglia et al., "The association of soy food consumption with the risk of subtype of breast cancers defined by hormone receptor and HER2 status", *International Journal of Cancer*, vol. 139, no. 4, pp. 742-748, 2016. Available: https://pubmed.ncbi.nlm.nih.gov/27038352/. [Accessed 27 April 2020].

[464] Y. Yu, X. Jing, H. Li, X. Zhao and D. Wang, "Soy isoflavone consumption and colorectal cancer risk: a systematic review and meta-analysis", *Scientific Reports*, vol. 6, no. 1, 2016. Available: https://pubmed.ncbi.nlm.nih.gov/27170217/. [Accessed 27 April 2020].

[465] G. Tse and G. Eslick, "Soy and isoflavone consumption and risk of gastrointestinal cancer: a systematic review and meta-analysis", *European Journal of Nutrition*, vol. 55, no. 1, pp.

63-73, 2014. Available: https://pubmed.ncbi.nlm.nih.gov/25547973/. [Accessed 27 April 2020].

[466] "Spinach, raw Nutrition Facts & Calories", *Nutritiondata.self.com*. [Online]. Available: https://nutritiondata.self.com/facts/vegetables-and-vegetable-products/2626/2. [Accessed: 26- Apr- 2020].

[467] "Countries by Spinach Production", *AtlasBig*, 2018. [Online]. Available: https://www.atlasbig.com/en-gb/countries-by-spinach-production#. [Accessed: 14- Jun- 2020].

[468] "Blue-Green Algae: MedlinePlus Supplements", *Medlineplus.gov*, 2019. [Online]. Available: https://medlineplus.gov/druginfo/natural/923.html. [Accessed: 26- Apr- 2020].

[469] P. Karkos, S. Leong, C. Karkos, N. Sivaji and D. Assimakopoulos, "Spirulinain Clinical Practice: Evidence-Based Human Applications", *Evidence-Based Complementary and Alternative Medicine*, vol. 2011, pp. 1-4, 2011. Available: https://www.ncbi.nlm.nih.gov/pmc/articles/PMC3136577/. [Accessed 26 April 2020].

[470] M. Petruzzello, "stevia | Description, Plant, & Sweetener", *Encyclopedia Britannica*. [Online]. Available: https://www.britannica.com/plant/stevia-plant. [Accessed: 26- Apr- 2020].

[471] "St. John's wort Uses, Side Effects & Warnings - Drugs.com", *Drugs.com*, 2020. [Online]. Available: https://www.drugs.com/mtm/st-john-s-wort.html. [Accessed: 27- Jun- 2020].

[472] *Files.nccih.nih.gov*, 2015. [Online]. Available: https://files.nccih.nih.gov/s3fs-public/SJW_and_Depression_11-30-2015.pdf. [Accessed: 27- Jun- 2020].

[473] "Human Metabolome Database: Showing metabocard for Hyperforin (HMDB0030463)", *Hmdb.ca*, 2019. [Online]. Available: https://hmdb.ca/metabolites/HMDB0030463#enzymes. [Accessed: 04- Jan- 2022].

[474] R. Brasted, "sulfur | Definition, Properties, Uses, & Facts", *Encyclopedia Britannica*, 2020. [Online]. Available: https://www.britannica.com/science/sulfur. [Accessed: 28- Apr- 2020].

[475] A. Stimola, *Sulfur*. New York: Rosen Central, 2008, p. 6.

[476] P. S, "Sulfur in Human Nutrition and Applications in Medicine", *PubMed*, 2002. [Online]. Available: https://pubmed.ncbi.nlm.nih.gov/11896744/. [Accessed: 28- Apr- 2020].

[477] J. Brosnan and M. Brosnan, "The Sulfur-Containing Amino Acids: An Overview", *The Journal of Nutrition*, vol. 136, no. 6, pp. 1636S-1640S, 2006. Available: https://academic.oup.com/jn/article/136/6/1636S/4664439. [Accessed 15 June 2020].

[478] M. Nimni, B. Han and F. Cordoba, "Are we getting enough sulfur in our diet?", *Nutrition & Metabolism*, vol. 4, no. 1, p. 24, 2007. Available: https://www.ncbi.nlm.nih.gov/pmc/articles/PMC2198910/. [Accessed 28 April 2020].

[479] Z. POLOSKY, *21ST CENTURY HOMESTEAD*. [Place of publication not identified]: LULU COM, 2015, p. 146.

[480] "Plants Profile for Tanacetum vulgare (common tansy)", *Plants.usda.gov*. [Online]. Available: https://plants.usda.gov/core/profile?symbol=TAVU. [Accessed: 20- May- 2020].

[481] O. Panasiuk, "Response of Colorado potato beetles,Leptinotarsa decemlineata (Say), to volatile components of tansy,Tanacetum vulgare", *Journal of Chemical Ecology*, vol. 10, no. 9, pp.

1325-1333, 1984. Available: https://pubmed.ncbi.nlm.nih.gov/24317584/. [Accessed 16 June 2020].

[482] L. Sablon, J. Dickens, É. Haubruge and F. Verheggen, "Chemical Ecology of the Colorado Potato Beetle, Leptinotarsa decemlineata (Say) (Coleoptera: Chrysomelidae), and Potential for Alternative Control Methods", *Insects*, vol. 4, no. 1, pp. 31-54, 2012. Available: https://www.ncbi.nlm.nih.gov/pmc/articles/PMC4553428/. [Accessed 16 June 2020].

[483] M. Poll, "Ti Tree oil, an ancient Bundjulung medicine", *Medium*, 2015. [Online]. Available: https://medium.com/@mattpoll2/ti-tree-oil-an-ancient-bundjulung-medicine-8c74ad526171. [Accessed: 12- Nov- 2021].

[484] Nccih.nih.gov, 2016. [Online]. Available: https://www.nccih.nih.gov/health/tea-tree-oil. [Accessed: 26- May- 2020].

[485] "A Brief History of Thyme", *HISTORY*, 2020. [Online]. Available: https://www.history.com/news/a-brief-history-of-thyme#. [Accessed: 17- Jun- 2020].

[486] "Thymol", *Pubchem.ncbi.nlm.nih.gov*, 2020. [Online]. Available: https://pubchem.ncbi.nlm.nih.gov/compound/6989. [Accessed: 12- Nov- 2021].

[487] I. Mozos, D. Stoian, A. Caraba, C. Malainer, J. Horbańczuk and A. Atanasov, "Lycopene and Vascular Health", *Frontiers in Pharmacology*, vol. 9, 2018. Available: https://www.ncbi.nlm.nih.gov/pmc/articles/PMC5974099/. [Accessed 29 April 2020].

[488] S. Prasad, A. Tyagi and B. Aggarwal, "Recent Developments in Delivery, Bioavailability, Absorption and Metabolism of Curcumin: the Golden Pigment from Golden Spice", *Cancer Research and Treatment*, vol. 46, no. 1, pp. 2-18, 2014. Available: https://www.e-crt.org/journal/view.php?doi=10.4143/crt.2014.46.1.2. [Accessed 17 June 2020].

[489] S. Prasad and B. Aggarwal, "Chapter 13. Turmeric, the Golden Spice.", *Ncbi.nlm.nih.gov*, 2011. [Online]. Available: https://www.ncbi.nlm.nih.gov/books/NBK92752/. [Accessed: 29- Apr- 2020].

[490] J. Hellson, *Ethnobotany of the Blackfoot Indians*. Ottawa: National Museums of Canada, 1974, p. 101. [Accessed: 29- Apr- 2020].

[491] "Uva Ursi Uses, Benefits & Dosage - Drugs.com Herbal Database", *Drugs.com*, 2020. [Online]. Available: https://www.drugs.com/npp/uva-ursi.html. [Accessed: 12- Nov- 2021].

[492] J. Horn and R. Miller, *The smart woman's guide to midlife and beyond*. Oakland, CA: New Harbinger Publications, 2008, pp. 229 & 230.

[493] *Nccih.nih.gov*, 2016. [Online]. Available: https://www.nccih.nih.gov/health/valerian. [Accessed: 20- May- 2020].

[494] L. Chevalier de Jaucourt, "Vanilla", *Quod.lib.umich.edu*, 1765. [Online]. Available: https://quod.lib.umich.edu/d/did/did2222.0000.830. [Accessed: 29- Apr- 2020].

[495] B. Shyamala, M. Naidu, G. Sulochanamma and P. Srinivas, "Studies on the Antioxidant Activities of Natural Vanilla Extract and Its Constituent Compounds through in-Vitro Models", *Journal of Agricultural and Food Chemistry*, vol. 55, no. 19, pp. 7738-7743, 2007. Available:

https://pubmed.ncbi.nlm.nih.gov/17715988/. [Accessed 29 April 2020].

[496] "Vervain Uses, Benefits & Dosage - Drugs.com Herbal Database", *Drugs.com*, 2020. [Online]. Available: https://www.drugs.com/npp/vervain.html. [Accessed: 18- Jun- 2020].

[497] "Wintergreen: Uses, Side Effects, Interactions, Dosage, and Warning", *Webmd.com*, 2020. [Online]. Available: https://www.webmd.com/vitamins/ai/ingredientmono-783/wintergreen. [Accessed: 07- Dec- 2021].

[498] *Bonap.net*, 2014. [Online]. Available: http://bonap.net/MapGallery/County/Galium%20odoratum.png. [Accessed: 18- Jun- 2020].

[499] P. Perkins-Veazie, J. Collins, A. Davis and W. Roberts, "Carotenoid Content of 50 Watermelon Cultivars", *Journal of Agricultural and Food Chemistry*, vol. 54, no. 7, pp. 2593-2597, 2006. Available: https://pubmed.ncbi.nlm.nih.gov/16569049/. [Accessed 24 April 2020].

[500] M. Rodriguez-Concepcion et al., "A global perspective on carotenoids: Metabolism, biotechnology, and benefits for nutrition and health", *Progress in Lipid Research*, vol. 70, pp. 62-93, 2018. Available: https://www.sciencedirect.com/science/article/abs/pii/S0163782717300395. [Accessed 24 April 2020].

[501] 2017. [Online]. Available: https://www.wildflower.org/plants/result.php?id_plant=ACMI2. [Accessed: 07- Dec- 2021].

[502] C. Oellig, J. Schunck and W. Schwack, "Determination of caffeine, theobromine and theophylline in Mate beer and Mate soft drinks by high-performance thin-layer chromatography", *Journal of Chromatography A*, vol. 1533, pp. 208-212, 2018. Available: https://pubmed.ncbi.nlm.nih.gov/29241955/. [Accessed 04 January 2022].

[503] A. Gambero and M. Ribeiro, "The Positive Effects of Yerba Maté (Ilex paraguariensis) in Obesity", *Nutrients*, vol. 7, no. 2, pp. 730-750, 2015. Available: https://www.ncbi.nlm.nih.gov/pmc/articles/PMC4344557/. [Accessed 19 June 2020].

[504] D. Loria, E. Barrios and R. Zanetti, "Cancer and yerba mate consumption: a review of possible associations", *Revista Panamericana de Salud Pública*, vol. 25, no. 6, pp. 530-539, 2009. Available: https://pubmed.ncbi.nlm.nih.gov/19695149/. [Accessed 7 Dec 2021].

[505] *Nccih.nih.gov*, 2016. [Online]. Available: https://www.nccih.nih.gov/health/yohimbe. [Accessed: 26- May- 2020].

[506] T. Kearney, N. Tu and C. Haller, "Adverse Drug Events Associated with Yohimbine-Containing Products: A Retrospective Review of the California Poison Control System Reported Cases", *Annals of Pharmacotherapy*, vol. 44, no. 6, pp. 1022-1029, 2010. Available: https://pubmed.ncbi.nlm.nih.gov/20442348/. [Accessed 26 May 2020].

[507] https://www.ncbi.nlm.nih.gov/pubmed/8083574?dopt=Abstract (Downloaded 4th May 2020)

[508] R. Caruso, "Why does it take so long for our vision to adjust to a darkened theater after we come in from bright sunlight?", *Scientific American*, 2007. [Online]. Available: https://www.scientificamerican.com/article/experts-eyes-adjust-to-darkness/. [Accessed:

20- Jun- 2020].

[509] A. Wise, "Phytate and zinc bioavailability", *International Journal of Food Sciences and Nutrition*, vol. 46, no. 1, pp. 53-63, 1995. Available: https://pubmed.ncbi.nlm.nih.gov/7712343/. [Accessed 7 Dec 2021].

[510] K. Hambidge, L. Miller, J. Westcott, X. Sheng and N. Krebs, "Zinc bioavailability and homeostasis", *The American Journal of Clinical Nutrition*, vol. 91, no. 5, pp. 1478S-1483S, 2010. Available: https://www.ncbi.nlm.nih.gov/pmc/articles/PMC2854914/. [Accessed 4 May 2020].

[511] "Office of Dietary Supplements - Zinc", *Ods.od.nih.gov*, 2020. [Online]. Available: https://ods.od.nih.gov/factsheets/Zinc-HealthProfessional/. [Accessed: 04- May- 2020].

[512] E. Menzano and P. Carlen, "Zinc Deficiency and Corticosteroids in the Pathogenesis of Alcoholic Brain Dysfunction-A Review", *Alcoholism: Clinical and Experimental Research*, vol. 18, no. 4, pp. 895-901, 1994. Available: https://pubmed.ncbi.nlm.nih.gov/7978102/. [Accessed 4 May 2020].

[513] "Office of Dietary Supplements - Zinc", *Ods.od.nih.gov*, 2020. [Online]. Available: https://ods.od.nih.gov/factsheets/Zinc-HealthProfessional/. [Accessed: 04- May- 2020].

[514] "NLM Herb Garden", *Nlm.nih.gov*, 2019. [Online]. Available: https://www.nlm.nih.gov/about/herbgarden/index.html. [Accessed: 09- May- 2020].

[515] "Herbs and Supplements: MedlinePlus", *Medlineplus.gov*, 2020. [Online]. Available: https://medlineplus.gov/druginfo/herb_All.html. [Accessed: 09- May- 2020].

[516] R. Scheer and D. Moss, "Dirt Poor: Have Fruits and Vegetables Become Less Nutritious?", *Scientific American*, 2011. [Online]. Available: https://www.scientificamerican.com/article/soil-depletion-and-nutrition-loss/. [Accessed: 09- May- 2020].

[517] A. Serpen, V. Gökmen and V. Fogliano, "Total antioxidant capacities of raw and cooked meats", *Meat Science*, vol. 90, no. 1, pp. 60-65, 2012. Available: https://pubmed.ncbi.nlm.nih.gov/21684086/. [Accessed 20 June 2020].

[518] R. Carmody and R. Wrangham, "Cooking and the Human Commitment to a High-quality Diet", *Cold Spring Harbor Symposia on Quantitative Biology*, vol. 74, no. 0, pp. 427-434, 2009. Available: https://pubmed.ncbi.nlm.nih.gov/19843593/. [Accessed 20 June 2020].

[519] P. Evenepoel, B. Geypens, A. Luypaerts, M. Hiele, Y. Ghoos and P. Rutgeerts, "Digestibility of Cooked and Raw Egg Protein in Humans as Assessed by Stable Isotope Techniques", *The Journal of Nutrition*, vol. 128, no. 10, pp. 1716-1722, 1998. Available: https://pubmed.ncbi.nlm.nih.gov/9772141/. [Accessed 20 June 2020].

[520] M. Kimura and Y. Itokawa, "Cooking Losses of Minerals in Foods and Its Nutritional Significance", *PubMed*, 1990. [Online]. Available: https://pubmed.ncbi.nlm.nih.gov/2081985/. [Accessed: 20- Jun- 2020].

[521] "TNAU Agritech Portal :: Sustainable Agriculture", *Agritech.tnau.ac.in*, 2015. [Online]. Available: http://agritech.tnau.ac.in/nutrition/nutri_cookingtips_nutrientloss.html. [Accessed: 15- Dec- 2021].

[522] C. McClain, V. Vatsalya and M. Cave, "Role of Zinc in the Development/Progression of Alcoholic Liver Disease", *Current Treatment Options in Gastroenterology*, vol. 15, no. 2, pp. 285-295, 2017. Available: https://www.ncbi.nlm.nih.gov/pmc/articles/PMC6206836/. [Accessed 20 June 2020].

[523] "Alcohol and Nutrition - Alcohol Alert No. 22- 1993", *Pubs.niaaa.nih.gov*, 2000. [Online]. Available: https://pubs.niaaa.nih.gov/publications/aa22.htm. [Accessed: 09- May- 2020].

[524] S. Barve, S. Chen, I. Kirpich, W. Watson and C. McClain, "Development, Prevention, and Treatment of Alcohol-Induced Organ Injury: The Role of Nutrition", *PubMed Central (PMC)*, 2017. [Online]. Available: https://www.ncbi.nlm.nih.gov/pmc/articles/PMC5513692/. [Accessed: 09- May- 2020].

[525] T. Morck, S. Lynch and J. Cook, "Inhibition of food iron absorption by coffee", *The American Journal of Clinical Nutrition*, vol. 37, no. 3, pp. 416-420, 1983. Available: https://pubmed.ncbi.nlm.nih.gov/6402915/. [Accessed 17 Dec 2021].

[526] H. Hoffman, R. Phyliky and C. Fleming, *Gastrojournal.org*, 1988. [Online]. Available: https://www.gastrojournal.org/article/0016-5085(88)90445-3/pdf. [Accessed: 09- May- 2020].

[527] B. Lönnerdal, "Dietary Factors Influencing Zinc Absorption", *The Journal of Nutrition*, vol. 130, no. 5, pp. 1378S-1383S, 2000. Available: https://pubmed.ncbi.nlm.nih.gov/10801947/. [Accessed 9 May 2020].

[528] G. Cizza and K. Rother, "Was Feuerbach right: are we what we eat?", *Journal of Clinical Investigation*, vol. 121, no. 8, pp. 2969-2971, 2011. Available: https://www.ncbi.nlm.nih.gov/pmc/articles/PMC3148750/ [Accessed 6 May 2021].

Printed in Great Britain
by Amazon